*A guide for recovering wholeness in
body, mind, and spirit.*

YOU
CAN HELP
WITH YOUR
HEALING

VERNON J. BITTNER

AUGSBURG Publishing House • Minneapolis

To
all who are broken
and are seeking recovery

Contents

Preface

THE THOUGHTS AND IDEAS RECORDED in this book are based on experiences in my life and the lives of those I have met. These events give witness to my journey toward healing. "Healing" is a fascinating word. Often we think of it in terms of cure. However, there is no such thing as a cure for the human condition or the human dilemma. Every one of us will eventually die. Therefore when we think of healing, we need to think of it in the Judeo-Christian tradition which equates it with salvation, or being made whole. Being made whole or finding salvation, however, does not only pertain to one's spiritual life, but to one's emotional and physical life as well. It is concerned with the recovery of the proper balance of one's body, mind, and spirit.

This holistic view of healing and recovery is supported by many in the medical profession. For some time most physicians have emphasized the bodily aspects of illness.

The difficulty with this is that the doctor's attention is distracted from the emotional and spiritual aspects of that illness. There have been all kinds of studies and cases which show that people do not get well if they do not want to get well. This is true of physical illness as well as emotional and spiritual sicknesses.

For example, diabetic patients, while being treated physically for their problem, have died. People have died in surgery, not because of a slip of the knife, but because they believed they were going to die. Dialysis patients have died because they believed there was no hope. Patients being treated in intensive care units have died because of the crisis atmosphere, turmoil, and isolation they experienced in that unit, in spite of the technical advantages available for them physically. Some of these people died because they felt unloved, faithless, hopeless, and isolated. They lacked the spiritual gifts of self-esteem, faith, hope, and love. They could see no healing possible for them. It's as though they chose the only alternative they could find.

There are also people who do not recover from illness because they do not take any responsibility for their recovery. It is estimated that more than 50% of those who consult a doctor do not even follow their doctor's recommendations. Instead of taking responsibility for their lives and their health, they are making the doctor responsible. They too believe, as many doctors still believe, that illness and healing are exclusively physical. And if health only involves the physical, they think they have no responsibility for their health. People will only take responsibility for their illness when they accept the fact that their health is also dependent on their emotional and spiritual condition. In addition, they need to accept that their primary illness may not be physical at all, but may be emotional or spiritual, or a combination of these.

Three patients were undergoing surgery for detached retina. They were each given a test to determine their acceptance of their situation. The person who scored the highest got well faster than those who did not have such an "expectant faith."

There are many examples of the healing that takes place when patients possess expectant faith, such as 176 well-authenticated cases of cancer which were remitted without treatment, confirmed by two surgeons' reports. Conversely there is also evidence that depression inhibits the immune system of the body and that persons with certain types of personality disorders are prone to develop various illnesses shortly after a personal loss.

Assuming this to be true, some physicians believe that opposite emotions such as love instead of anger (depression is anger turned inward), faith instead of unbelief, and hope instead of hopelessness could retard the spread of cancer because these attitudes would stimulate the immune responses of the body.

Logically, then, our healing involves considering the person holistically. Recovery from illness involves our wanting to get well, as well as taking responsibility for the process. Whether or not we want to get well and take responsibility for our healing is mainly determined by our attitude toward life. These attitudes are primarily spiritual in nature. Anger is overcome by forgiveness because we have been forgiven; devaluating the self is overcome by love because of God's love for us; unbelief and hopelessness are overcome by a faith and a hope in something beyond ourselves.

Therefore, when I speak of healing and recovery, I

speak from the conviction that this does not happen unless we have tapped the spiritual part of ourselves—unless we are spiritually whole. Therefore, healing—the healing of the total person—is a result of spiritual recovery. Admittedly, perfect healing or recovery is not possible in this life—only in the life to come with Christ, because all of us will get sick and die some day and none of us will attain *perfect* wholeness physically, emotionally, or spiritually. But healing or recovery will not occur without spiritual recovery—without the spiritual gifts of faith, hope, and love.

I am convinced that healing or spiritual recovery can not be discussed in general terms. It can only be talked about personally. Therefore, the only spiritual recovery that I can talk about is my own and that of others I've met. In this book I speak of my blindness in accepting my illness, my unwillingness to take responsibility for my recovery, and my sick desire to prescribe for my recovery without the need of God. I talk of my resentment toward God, my parents, and myself. Here is my need for love, acceptance, and forgiveness. Here are things that I am still working at to change wherever I can and accept whatever I can't change, so that each day has some moments of power, love, peace, and joy. I only hope that my sharing will be an aid in helping you along your way, because none of us has "arrived."

I hope we will all continue to work at our own healing or spiritual recovery; otherwise our lives could well be boring and empty, sick and sinful, destructive and suicidal.

Spiritual recovery is a process of maturing both mentally and spiritually, so that healing can take place. This includes growing in our relationship with God, with others, and with ourselves.

In this book, I am using the Twelve Steps of Recovery as used in Alcoholics Anonymous as an outline for the process of spiritual recovery. I am using these twelve steps not only because they are based on the principles found in the Bible, but also because they have been applied to other self-help groups like Emotions Anonymous, Overeaters Anonymous, as well as Al-Anon, Alateens, and Pre-Alateens, which are organizations for family members of the alcoholic. Here I am adapting the twelve steps primarily to the Christian faith in hopes that it will help those of the Christian persuasion to have a more concrete guide for spiritual recovery.

The first step in the recovery program is to admit that you are not able to control a lot of things in life and that you are not able to manage anyone else's life either. The second and third steps have to do with acknowledging a need for God and turning your will and life over to him. The fourth and tenth steps encourage us to realize the importance of being aware of our strengths and weaknesses through the process of a daily personal inventory, so that we don't foolishly harbor any wrongs against ourselves, God, or others. The fifth step is to make confession to ourselves, to God, and to another person we trust, in order to more fully experience the joy of forgiveness. The sixth and seventh steps help us to be open enough to God to allow him to remove the destructive aspects of our personalities so that we can make our personality traits more constructive. The eighth and ninth steps encourage us to be aware of those people with whom we need to be reconciled and actively pursue restoration of harmonious relationships. The eleventh step reminds us of our need to stay in touch with God through prayer and meditation so that we may seek to know his will for our lives and have the power to fulfill his will in our lives. The twelfth step is the challenge to share the joy and serenity of our spiritual rebirth also with others so that they might know that there is hope for them as well.

Many have found that if these principles are practiced as a way of life, they can give people the strength, courage, and wisdom to live happier, more productive lives. However, the purpose of this life-style goes beyond finding a happy, serene life. I am convinced that this way of life will give people the necessary tools to take responsibility for their own health and wholeness. It will show them how they can work at their own spiritual recovery.

The result of this spiritual recovery is not only that we feel deeply moved, sometimes to the point of tears, but also uplifted with a tremendous feeling of exhilaration. Feelings are not the only measure of the nearness of God.

Feelings by themselves are not enough. Sometimes we have to act as if we feel uplifted whether we do or not. Because there will be days in which we will feel awed and moved; other days when the sky will be as grey as it ever was and the glory will have passed away. Then we may be filled with the curious suspicion that religion is a chemical which only gives temporary relief.

Spiritual recovery is like love between a man and a woman. Even though they may love each other very dearly, they will not always feel that love. Life is never one long honeymoon. With most marriages there are times when those involved may be asking themselves whether or not they do love each other. Here they are making the same mistake in regard to love as many make about their spiritual life. They are judging whether they love each other by how they feel. But let someone say something untrue about the other person and they will immediately come to the other's defense. Their love was there all the time, but it was dormant.

Those who are on the way toward spiritual recovery have something in addition to feelings to indicate their progress. First, they have a changed attitude toward life. Instead of being hostile, cynical, guilty, or afraid, they have a new sense of love, joy, peace, and power.

In addition, those whose lives are being renewed become highly motivated toward accomplishing their goals in life. They also have a trust and a love for others, a desire to grow in understanding of God's will for their lives, and an eagerness to share what they have found with others. With God's help they find the strength to change what they can, the courage to accept what they cannot change, and the wisdom to know the difference. With God's help they can help with their healing.

But we must also remember that there may be days when our lives will show none of these changes. We may have no deep desires or uplifted feelings. When that happens, we must continue to reach out for God's hand-- believing that he wants us more than we want him, he trusts us more than we trust him, and he loves us more than we will ever love him. Otherwise we will not find the serenity, strength, courage, and wisdom we need for spiritual recovery. If we let our wonder-filled quest for spiritual recovery slip away from us, we will not only deprive others of our gifts, but we will not help with our healing and wholeness. Spending eternity with God is a gift that we cannot earn. But the salvation that Jesus talks about is both in the future and in the present, and it means being healed spiritually, emotionally, and physically. Throughout the New Testament Jesus equates healing and salvation, and his concern for us is that we experience the joy of salvation (spiritual recovery) here on earth, too.

1 Do You Want to Be Healed?

For I do not do the good I want, but the evil I do not want is what I do.   Romans 7:19

MY NAME IS VERN BITTNER, and I am a self-destructor. I want you to notice that I didn't say I am alcoholic or abusing myself with any other chemicals, or that I go off the deep end in fanatic religiosity. There are a lot of ways to destroy one's self other than chemical abuse. There are some people who are "workaholics" or "foodaholics." There are other people who are controlled by their emotional and religious attitudes and become either mentally or physically ill. Essentially, anyone who abuses himself physically, emotionally, or spiritually is a self-destructor. But the method by which I tried to destroy myself was to actually attempt suicide. This occurred more than twenty years ago.

During this period of my life, I did not see that my life was of much value, even though I was constantly trying to prove my worth to myself and others. I was really a nice guy and that was a big part of the problem. I was so nice I could not say no to anyone. My involvement with people was at a very immature level—either they were using me or I was using them. When that did not work or I became tired of it, I would have to lie to get out of the "no win" situations in which I found myself.

The obvious result of this behavior was alienation, not only from those with whom I had a superficial relationship, but also from those who loved me. This isolation from people was also accompanied by my separation from God. When people feel distant, God seems distant, too.

I found myself all alone and there seemed to be no solution to my problem. No matter how I tried to unravel the patterns I was used to, it did not work. Somehow, I had never learned how to have healthy, mature relationships with people.

My feeling of isolation was heightened by my self-hatred and self-pity, and by the resulting depression. Those were dark, hopeless days—days of suspicion and unbelief. My life was out of my control. I was governed by all that was evil and destructive in myself. It seemed that only my destruction would give me relief.

My most serious suicide attempt came in the spring of the year. Oh, there had been other feeble attempts, but this was serious. I hadn't threatened to do it this time. I had not told anyone about it. It was the Saturday night prior to Easter Sunday. Perhaps in my sick mind this was an unconscious attempt to defy God because I felt he had forsaken me. Why should I have any hope—let alone the hope of the resurrection? After all, what had he done for me, except abandon me, and leave me hopelessly out of control?

The truth was that God had not isolated himself from me, I had separated myself from him—partly by my behavior and partly by my warped understanding of him. I did not see him as a God of love and forgiveness, but only as a God of wrath. My human experience had led me to believe that he wouldn't understand, and also to think that I had nothing to do with my hopeless condition.

I knew that there was a train at 9:45 P.M. I was determined to let it do the work—I was sure that this would be a quick way to die. The engineer would either not see me or he would be unable to stop in time even if he did see something on the track. I placed myself where there would be no question about whether I would die. I was sure I would be decapitated. I had convinced myself that it took more courage to kill myself than to live. This, of course, is never true, but I wasn't thinking straight. My life had become unmanageable.

I could see the train's light as it came down the track. The closer it came the more I was convinced that this was the only thing I could do. Hadn't I tried everything else? Wasn't my life hopeless? Had not even God forsaken me?

Just as the train was about to separate my head from my body, there was a power greater than my will to die that literally catapulted me from the track. When the train had passed and my heart began to beat again, I found myself on the opposite side from which I had begun. Yes, I was still alive. I had not died. But why?

My first reaction was anger and disgust with myself. What a miserable excuse of a man—couldn't I even do that right? I had even failed at destroying myself.

I got up, brushed myself off, and began to walk. I was overwhelmed by the thought of still being alive and wondering why I was not killed. And then it struck me. God had not wanted me to die. God had a purpose for my life. But unless I was willing to admit that my life was unmanageable, I would continue to be powerless over my destructive attitude. If this did not change, I *would* kill myself. If it was not by suicide, then it would probably be by some other conscious or subconscious way.

As I look back on this experience, I am reminded of the account of Jesus' healing of the invalid beside the pool of Bethesda (John 5:2-15). This invalid had to admit his inability to control his life and the environment around him. For thirty-eight years he had been trying to get others to be responsible for him and his illness. He was constantly preoccupied with the thought of how he could get others to help him. But Jesus knew that the man had to help himself. Healing would occur only when he took responsibility for his own illness. He had to admit that he was powerless to control the people around him and make them responsible for his healing. He had to make the decision of whether or not he really wanted to get well. If he did want to be well, then he would have to be responsible for the healing process, either by being open to the healing power of God or by drawing on God's strength to help him change his attitude so that he would be willing to accept his condition and not make others responsible for it.

The significant issue in the invalid's healing (and in the healing of anyone for that matter) is whether or not we stop trying to make others responsible for our illness. We must admit that we are responsible for coping with our illness, and that we are powerless over whether or not we have it. This, however, does not mean that we are powerless over any healing, because sometimes people become temporarily healed in spite of themselves. But healing will not take place unless one accepts his or her illness.

Her life was unmanageable

As a hospital chaplain who is involved in the healing process, I am aware that illness can make people feel out of control. Being sick is one of the things that can make a person's life seem unmanageable. Edna was in her late thirties—a rather small, wiry woman with a great deal of determination. But she was a person who had never had a very good opinion of herself. She always felt that she had to prove herself to herself and others by doing things for them. Working for her family had given her life meaning. I had known her more than three years. A few years earlier multiple sclerosis had been diagnosed. At first she functioned normally, but as time went on there were more and more things that she could not do. She was devastated by her illness, because she had always found her value as a person in what she could do for others. The more she found she could not do or do well, the more depressed, despondent, and hopeless she became. During the first two years of her illness she attempted suicide twice. A year ago her husband and her psychiatrist had become so concerned that they wanted to put her in a nursing home for her own protection, not because she could not take care of herself, but because she would not. She had also allowed her physical condition to deteriorate and consequently she had lost much of her mobility, now barely creeping along with the aid of a walker.

The only thing that prevented her from going to a nursing home was the disagreement between her general practitioner and her psychiatrist about the plans for her treatment. During this indecision she was able to convince her personal physician that she should come to see me. She had met me during her hospitalization for depression.

She had come to trust me, and also she felt that going into counseling was one way she could get her husband and the psychiatrist to stop talking about putting her in a nursing home. Admittedly, her motivation for getting well was not the best—but then, who always does things for the right motive?

I began seeing her and her husband every week. She seemed to be making progress, so I started to see her every other week. She was functioning at home as well as she could—considering her condition. Soon I suggested that she come every three or four weeks. It was then that things began to fall apart. She became despondent, resentful, and preoccupied again because she did not feel appreciated by her family and she needed outside support more frequently. I thought we had worked through her unwillingness to accept her illness, her resentment about all the things she could not do, her feelings of worthlessness (because her value as a person was based on what she could do for others), and her incurable condition. But she would have to change her attitude regarding multiple sclerosis (with God's help) if she wanted to be healed.

I went to my office at the hospital a couple of hours before Edna's appointment. A few minutes after I arrived a call came from Edna's sister. Her voice was noticeably anxious and concerned. She had seen Edna last week and was worried about her attitude. "She seemed so bitter and even somewhat paranoid. She accused me of not believing that she could handle things at home—and I never said that. I thought you ought to know that she thinks everyone is against her. I just don't know what to do!"

I thanked her for calling me. We talked for awhile and came to the conclusion that we should not play any games with her. Rather, Edna should be confronted about this behavior. She agreed to come to my office for Edna's appointment so that we could confront her together about what she was doing to herself.

When Edna arrived she was surprised to see her sister and even more surprised when I asked them to come into my office together. I asked Edna's sister to tell her what she had told me. I was convinced that the main problem was her unwillingness to admit that she could not control her illness. In spite of all of my efforts and everyone else's, she still had not accepted that she was powerless over her illness. She was trying to solve her problem by refusing to face it; she thought she could bury it. She refused to accept responsibility for her attitudes. She was not being healed emotionally or spiritually because she would not accept that she was powerless over her physical condition.

Edna's sister told her how worried she was because Edna only listened to what she wanted to hear. Edna had believed that she was of no value at home, and she was so convinced it was true that she had misinterpreted what her sister had said.

I asked Edna if she would like to accept the fact that she could not control, change, or cure her illness. I told her she was using all of her energy to prove she did not have MS. Unless she stopped doing this she would not have any energy left to work on healing her emotional and spiritual attitudes.

"What do you want me to do—give up and die?" She began to cry. I told her that I did not want her to give up, but unless she accepted her illness her life would be hopeless. She first needed emotional and spiritual health so that she could live with her illness. Edna's MS would never get any better.

I told her I wanted to hear her say: "I will accept my

illness." She only responded to this by telling me she was not going to be a phony, and then she promptly changed the subject by telling me how unfeeling I was and that I did not really understand how hard it was for her. Again I asked her to say: "I will accept my illness." She protested once more and told me that she would, if she just knew how. I informed her that the *how* is making a commitment to *do* it. It is wanting to accept the reality of her illness.

She said: "I . . . I will accept it, . . . but it is so hard to do." I asked her if she understood what she had said to me. I told her that she had just told me: "Yes, I will, but no, I *won't*." I told her she was trying to con me and I did not appreciate that.

"Will you say: 'I will accept my illness'?" There was a long pause. Finally she said it. I asked her how she felt about saying it. She told me that it was scary, but right now she felt relieved because she had finally said it.

That was a difficult experience for Edna, her sister, and myself. But it was the turning point for Edna. It had taken more than two years for her to let go and admit that she had no control over her illness. Because she had accepted her powerlessness over MS, she was able to begin to work on her spiritual and emotional recovery. She would probably never be cured of her illness, but there *was healing* for her destructive attitude.

Not only is Edna powerless over her illness—or should we say her humanness—but so is everyone else. Every human being has something in his life that makes his life unmanageable at times. Each person has an aspect of life over which he or she is powerless, if not in the present, then in the future. After all, everyone is powerless over death.

The reality of our powerlessness over a part of our living

and over our dying reminds me that even though I was created in the image of God—evil, sickness, and death have become a part of me. Even though we were created in God's image, we have the freedom to make moral choices. When we use this freedom to choose evil, our choice corrupts us and evil becomes part of us. So, we are both good and evil at the same time. At times, this tension within us becomes unbearable and we find ourselves plagued by indecision and weakness. We feel powerless to do what we want to do (Romans 7:18-19).

To deny this tension within us, this powerlessness, or this inability to manage our lives at all times, is only fooling ourselves—and emotional and spiritual recovery, which makes life happy and meaningful, does not come about through self-deception or the denial of the concept of original sin. Spiritual recovery begins when we begin to accept our humanity with all of our assets and liabilities —that we are both sinner and saint. Otherwise we will be unable to help with our healing.

Lord, I want to be healed . . .
  But I want it to happen on my terms.

Lord, I want to be healed . . .
  But I don't want to admit I'm out of control.

Lord, I want to be healed . . .
  But I want to manage my own life.

Lord, I want to be healed . . .
  But I don't want to accept the limitations of my humanity.

Lord, I want to be healed.
  Help me to accept . . .
    my powerlessness,
    my unmanageability,

    my isolation, and
    my humanity,
So that healing can begin.

Lord, let it begin with me NOW!
Let me say: "Lord, I want to be healed!"

2 I'm Powerless

Hence I remind you to rekindle the gift of God that is within you through the laying on of my hands; for God did not give us a spirit of timidity but a spirit of power and love and self control.
2 Timothy 1:6-7

THAT SATURDAY NIGHT BEFORE EASTER had given me the opportunity to change my life. I believed that God had intervened in my life. God had taken my suicide attempt and turned it into a spiritual experience. Apparently I had to reach the depths of despair before I realized for the first time that I could not do anything to change my life by myself. No matter how hard I had tried or how many achievements I had accomplished, my life was a mess. If my life had continued as it was, I would have either killed myself or I would have become emotionally ill.

The longer I walked that evening the more convinced I became that God had not given me an irresolute, irrational, or irresponsible spirit; rather, he had given me a spirit of power, possibility, and purpose. However, until then I had not been aware of it.

I had known my sinful nature. I had known the power of evil within that kept telling me that I was no good, and that I was helpless and hopeless. However, I had not experienced that God had also created me *good*. I had forgotten the view of creation recorded in the book of Genesis that "God saw that it (creation) was good."

Unfortunately, I had needed an experience with death for me to realize how preoccupied (out of control) I was with my sinful nature, and how dead I was to the goodness and love of God within me. I began to realize that my wish to die was a tragedy. I became aware of how heartbreaking it was to wish I had never been born. I also discovered how I had wasted the love I had received from God at baptism by feeling powerless, hopeless, and helpless—instead of feeling that I belonged to God.

By realizing God's power I found that there was help and hope for my life. There was a solution for my resentment, loneliness, guilt, fear, procrastination, perfectionism, rejection of others, irresponsibility, lust, and greed. With God's power it would be possible to bring to life faith, hope, and love so that I could act in a realistic and responsible way.

I had come from the position of thinking I had faith in God to the realization that my faith had disappeared. I had gone through all of the motions of being a religious person. I followed all of the observances of the church. There was even a time within the structure of one denomination that I took the yearly pledge to neither smoke nor drink. I even kept it, but things did not seem to go any better. I was constantly asking for God's help, but my destructive ways continued, because I had not seen prayer primarily as a relationship with God.

Perhaps I had been deceiving myself all along. I was going through all of the right motions. I had even committed my life to God by deciding to study at the seminary, but the quality was not there. I had not really known the love and forgiveness of God in a personal way.

I had fooled myself into thinking I was humble, when I was really shy. I would "turn the other cheek," because I lacked the courage to stand for what I believed was right. I had wallowed in emotionalism and had mistaken it for a spiritual experience. My doing for others was really my attempt to do for myself. My religious activity was really my feeble attempt to avoid facing myself. In fact, nothing significantly religious would happen to me until I stopped trying to avoid my encounter with God. I had to make the decision to stop wanting to be religious to meet my own needs—to be honest enough to come clean so that God's grace could enter my life and give me some direction and purpose. I had not even prayed in the right manner. My prayers were always "give me this" or "give me that," instead of using prayer to establish an openness with God and man in order to love and be loved.

And my seminary experience . . . the more I think about it, the more I am convinced that it was my unconscious attempt to play God with people. I had deceived myself into thinking I was preparing to serve God. Instead, I was planning to be my own God. Thankfully, this did not last too long. My encounter with despair took care of that. As a result, I had to begin to look at how helpless I was, trying to be my own God. I began to see that I had to allow God to be in command or I would kill myself. I had to begin to see him not only as a power to be afraid of, but as a loving, forgiving force in my life that could transform me. All I had to do was to admit that I needed him, trust his promise to forgive, and desire to be open to his spirit within me. I needed to believe that there was hope for me . . . and God allowed me to see that.

God can't be found in serving others

As I write this, of course, I am also aware that not all of my motives were wrong. I did want the ministry because I thought it was the best way to help others. Unfortunately, helping others was a poor way to find a meaningful relationship with God. After all, who ever heard of "serve and you will find?" Before I could help others, I would have to know that there was a power in my life that could restore me to a life of maturity, love, and service. And before I could get that power for myself, I had to become aware of my need of God.

I think there are many people in the church who are like me—people who think they will find God by serving others. But who ever heard of sending people into the slums, or to work with those who are physically and emotionally ill, who have not yet experienced the power of God in their own lives? I am convinced that the demands would be too great. Without the power of that experience those people would lack the courage to stick to their commitment, or the strength not to get swallowed up by the very individuals they are seeking to help. You see, we who would find God by serving others are not really trying to find God anyway. Rather, *we are trying to be God ourselves.*

This does not mean that there is anything wrong in serving others. I am not criticizing the service given to those in need by people who have not experienced the power of God in their life. Certainly it is generous philanthropy even if it is not Christian service. But it is dangerous to tell someone that he will find God by serving others. My life is evidence of that. Unfortunately, the emphasis on "works" in my pietistic background partially resulted in my interpretation that God was found through service. In effect, I was trying to prescribe my own salvation without ever experiencing God's love and grace in my life.

God does not want our service as much as he wants us to experience the power of a relationship with him. Martha had the same problem (Luke 10:38-41). Somehow she thought she would find her relationship with her Lord by waiting on him and serving him, while her sister, Mary, spent her time sitting at the feet of Jesus listening to his teaching. We recall how upset Martha became with Mary. She even tried to convince Jesus that he ought to reprimand Mary for her lack of responsibility to the duties of the moment. But our Lord told Martha that she was pursuing the wrong things—her serving was only distracting her from meeting her Lord face to face. Jesus told Martha that Mary had made the choice to know her Lord on an intimate level and had found a relationship with him that would give her the power for her life that nothing could take from her.

How John came to believe

There are many people like Martha who never experience the power of God in their life. From outward appearances it seemed as though John had everything going his way. He was a handsome, middle-aged man and he was very successful. His wife was attractive as well, but she was more quiet and passive than her husband. Almost everyone who knew them felt that they made the ideal couple and certainly they were happily married if anyone was.

Both John and his wife were involved in the church.

John was not only active in men's groups in his own church but throughout the city. He was often asked to speak at other churches in the city, and had gained recognition as a religious writer.

But one September day the balloon burst. He called me in tears. His wife had told him she was going to leave him. He was able to convince his wife to come in for marriage counseling, but it was divorce counseling instead. There appeared to be too much hurt and resentment. John was unwilling to change his need to control his wife and stop his excessive activities in the church as well as the community. As a result, there was no forgiveness and no basis on which to begin working on their marriage.

Even the divorce didn't seem to change John's busyness. In fact, John became even more involved in church work. Now he was traveling throughout the country working for his church, in addition to holding down a full time job. This continued for about two years, until one day he collapsed at work. He was rushed to the hospital.

When I arrived in the room he was being fed intravenously. He was in pain, and so weak that he was having difficulty talking. The doctors were puzzled because they did not know the cause. And they were further confused by his extreme temperature.

I visited him daily but we did not talk at length until four days had passed. Then we talked about how he had brought on his own illness by allowing himself to get run down. He realized that he was being driven by something and unless he discovered what it was he would not be able to change his behavior.

As time went on he came to realize that his need to control his wife and everything around him, as well as his excessive work load, was all a result of the emptiness he felt. In spite of his involvement in the church and community he had never met his Lord face to face. He had been so busy running and doing that he had not discovered the power from God that is able to give a person the peace which passes all understanding.

John left the hospital knowing what he had to do. He discovered that he could not bring about his salvation by himself. He was going to have to believe that a power greater than himself would restore him to a life of peace and moderation.

John's recovery would happen only when he took the time to integrate God's power, love, and self-control into his life. I am not aware whether or not John has done this. The last time I talked to him, his pride was making it difficult for him to believe that all of his life he had been *serving* instead of *finding* his Lord.

Spiritual recovery means finding God's power, so that recovery can begin and you can help with your healing.

> Lord, I've been working so hard
>   to find your peace
> But all I've found is anxiety,
>   fear, and exhaustion.
> Somehow I was led to believe
>   that serving and helping . . . and working
>   were the most important.
> But I have only been deceiving myself
>   in order to make myself my own God.
>
> Lord, forgive me . . .
>   and help me.
> Help me to accept your love,
>   and integrate your power,
>   so that I can be in charge of my life,
>   instead of being controlled and driven
>   by the powerlessness I feel.

3 God,
Take Over

But seek first his kingdom and his righteousness,
and all these things shall be yours as well.
Matthew 6:33

FINDING GOD'S POWER and putting it to work in
your life are two different things. Putting
God's power to work, or appropriating that
power for your life, involves an act of the will.
You have to be willing to risk placing your life in God's
hands.

Many people believe in God, but yet have never turned
their lives over to him. The trouble with so many of us
is that we do not see God as he really is. For me, God had
seemed very punitive and legalistic. I did not think of him
as a god of love and forgiveness, who accepted me and
who would never desert me.

You would think that having gone through what I would
call my resurrection experience—moving from death to
new life—I would have no problem giving my life over
to God. It was obvious that I could not manage my life.
But turning my life over to God was not easy. Even
though, as I sat through the Easter sunrise service follow-

ing my attempted suicide, I realized that God really did love me. But I still found it hard to let God take over.

Turning one's life over to God, especially when we are insecure, is scary. As an insecure person, you already know you are not in charge of your own life and then you are supposed to give whatever little part of your life you have left to God. I had convinced myself that if I were to do that, I would not be an individual at all. Little did I know that the opposite was true. I would be able to find myself and be the person that God created me to be, if only I would allow God to give direction to my life. All I had to do to start that process in motion was to make the choice to be willing. Once I was willing to risk that, it began to happen. After all, what did I have to lose? Trying to run my life by myself had not worked. I might just as well turn it over to someone I could trust and who would not let me down.

There was still the fear that I would remain a dependent person if I turned my life over to God. Before, I had wanted God and others to take responsibility for my life. What would make a difference now?

But there was a difference. From here on, God would give me the courage to do things that I wanted others to do for me. He would be my strength when I felt weak and out of control. He would be the hope I needed to carry me through those situations which seemed to be impossible.

As I continued to progress in my willingness to turn my life over to God, I found that the rewards of happiness and peace of mind reinforced my behavior. Good results always help to encourage new behavior. The better the results the more willing I was to trust God's will for my life.

Yet perhaps the most difficult thing I had to learn was that I had not arrived. There were times when trusting

God to take over was too frightening, because I was afraid what God might expect me to do. But the consequences of this behavior, if I was willing to examine it, helped me to realize that I was not able to handle things by myself. I had limitations, just as every human being has.

The temptation of Jesus

As I think of the temptation of Jesus by the devil, in Luke 4:1-13, I am aware that Jesus used this experience as a guide for his own life. However, it is also a description of the choices that each person encounters who attempts to face life alone. (Right here I'd like you to take a moment to look at this passage in your Bible.) The freedom to make our own decisions is one of the significant aspects of the Christian faith. The important thing is that people establish the principles by which they will live, and the basic principle is to give their will and life over to the care of God. Just as this is a basic principle of the Christian faith, another basic principle is refusing to do only what is expedient.

The wilderness experience of Jesus in which he faced the three temptations of the devil was a very necessary part of the preparation for his life and ministry. It was his opportunity to clarify his priorities and directions. It was on this occasion that Jesus needed to know that his source of power was in being close to God, that his steadfastness was in his awareness of God's presence, and that the caring of his ministry was in his desire to find God. This is why he went to the desert, so that he could be alone with God.

Have you ever been in a desert alone at night? Have

you noticed how peaceful and quiet it is? Have you noticed how bright and close the stars seem to be? It is as if God has joined the heavens and earth before your very eyes and has made you a part of both. I am sure that this is why Jesus went to the desert. He knew that if he were alone, he would find God there.

In a sense we all need to have our own desert or wilderness experience. We need to have an opportunity to be with God—to define our goals and priorities for life—to turn our wills over to God.

Walking the deserted streets of Chicago early in the morning was my wilderness experience—or maybe it was the culmination of being in the "wilderness" for 25 years. For you it could be a walk in the woods, on the beach, or in the rain. It could be a retreat, a vacation, or the private altar in your home. It could be waking up early in the morning in a detoxification center, the intensive care unit of a hospital, or in your own bed with your spouse at your side.

The first temptation which Jesus faced, and which is common to all of us, was the temptation of allowing the pleasure principle to take over his life. He was tempted to satisfy his immediate sensual desire without thought about long-term goals. If you have ever been hungry, in pain, cold, or sexually aroused, you are aware of how these drives tend to block out all other interests.

I recall how easy it was for me to fall into the rut of saying what I thought people wanted to hear. I thought that if I would please people, then I could avoid the pain of rejection. Acceptance by others was so important to me because I had not accepted myself. Unfortunately, I found this behavior only avoided immediate pain and usually produced greater rejection and pain in the future.

There are all kinds of people in our society who live by this principle. About 75% of the marriage and family counseling that I do involves chemical dependency. All of these individuals are living by this principle. Alcohol or drugs are being used to avoid the immediate discomfort, whether physical, emotional, or spiritual.

One of the realizations that I came to during my own wilderness experience was that I had to start standing on my own two feet. I had to stop lying to others and to myself, because I realized that trying to please everyone ended up pleasing no one—not even myself. I had to begin to commit my life to a higher value. I had to turn my will and my life over to God. The only way that would happen was if I desired God's closeness and his presence in my life. No matter how hard it was for me to find God at times because of my defenses, I needed to be committed to making it happen. My desire alone would bring an added depth and meaning to my daily life. This is one aspect we all have to be more aware of and work hard at, because it is a constant temptation.

The second temptation Jesus encountered, and which all of us have, is to let our need for power take over our lives—to take personal ambition for prestige as the highest value in life. None of us is completely free of the desire at times to exploit others in order to better our own status.

One of the things that I still have trouble with is wanting to get others to do things for me—to push my responsibility off on someone else and in so doing take advantage of them. I remember that I would often use the excuse that I was weak, helpless, and hopeless. After all, what could anyone expect of someone like me? I would get people to feel sorry for me—even though I did realize that was a degrading attitude in itself—so that they would do it for me.

One of the unfortunate aspects of our culture today is that there are too many people who are taking advantage of others. I am convinced that there are two kinds of people in the world—the givers and the takers—and tragically, there are too many takers. Too many people today are living with the attitude that they will get the other person before that person gets them.

There are also a lot of people who feel that the way you get power and recognition is to seize it. You cannot get respect by seeking it; you get it by earning it.

We have all seen the person who wants the rewards without the work, the individual who wants the executive position without earning it. Power can never be demanded; rather it is the by-product of a dedicated life. Self-esteem and personal value grow out of one's commitment to help others.

This is the answer the devil gets from Jesus. He lets the devil know that the honored position is given to those who serve, in Matthew 20:26 and 27: "But whoever would be great among you must be your servant, and whoever would be first among you must be your slave." Status, according to Jesus, is found in having a meaningful relationship with God. It is a relationship that involves a life of service because of God's presence in our lives. If we are pleasing to God we are not only close to him, but we have received a power to live in a victorious way.

The third temptation, faced both by Jesus and by us, is to avoid responsibility for our lives. This is one of the alarming trends in our society. Many are excusing their present behavior by blaming it on a traumatic childhood, because of the poor parental relationships, or because of a lack of love.

I recall how I used my past as an excuse—sometimes consciously and sometimes unconsciously. After all, what could anyone expect from a person who had lost his mother early in life and who felt deserted by his father? I got a lot of mileage out of that one, but it only helped me to remain immature and isolated from God.

There are many people who are living a deterministic philosophy of life. This gives them an excuse for their present behavior. They are convinced that their past is controlling them and so "what will happen will happen." They deceive themselves into thinking this way in order to avoid changing the present.

Certainly, we need to be aware of our past and use it to understand our present behavior. But the past must not control or determine the present. Rather, we need to live responsibly in the present regardless of our past, incorporate the positive, and not be controlled by the negative. We also need to look toward the future, and use our past as a means of understanding it and guiding us in days to come.

Jesus took responsibility for his behavior in the wilderness as well as the choice he made following that experience. He did this because he had turned his life over to his Father. In doing this he set a pattern for his life and an example for us. If we follow this we will find the meaning, power, and strength to live a happy, productive life.

Do you really want him?

Spiritual recovery will never happen unless we have some time alone with God. But we will never find him unless we truly want him. The truth is that sometimes we want him and sometimes we don't. There is a conflict in our minds which can defeat our quest for God.

Certainly there are times when we truly long for God. There are times of loneliness, pain, and sorrow when we cry out for God's presence, comfort, and strength.

In fact, at these times we may even wonder where he is, because our pain and confusion close us off from God. When these times come we need to remember that our Lord wants to be close to us even more than we want him. He knows our pain because he endured the pain of the cross to bring about recovery, wholeness, and salvation.

During this time, our Lord longs to give us his presence, lift our spirits, steady our nerves, send his strength. Yes, there is no doubt that we want God at these times. We must have him or fall apart.

But also there are times when we do not want him. Many of us want God like we want an electric blanket— a little temporary comfort on a cold night, but then to be pushed away when the warmth of morning comes.

God is not like a magic genie who can be summoned to turn our garbage into gold and our slums into palaces. Nor must we bargain with him as Jacob did: "If God will be with me and keep me in this way that I go, and will give me bread to eat and clothing to wear, so that I come again to my father's house in peace, then the Lord shall be my God" (Genesis 28:20-21).

We must want him with our whole mind, for his own sake, and not for what we can get out of him.

When we find ourselves in this conflict we have to want his way more than our own way. Our need to be clean has to be greater than our need to want what we want when we want it. Our desire to be healed has to be more than our desire for power and prestige. We must seek his will more than we want to escape our responsibility to him and to ourselves.

We must desire him more than we desire anything else in the world. This is what it means to turn our wills and lives over to God. Turning our lives over to God means that we avoid the immediate pleasures for more worthwhile future goals, realize that power is not sought but caught, and accept responsibility for our own lives for the present and the future. Then we will promote our own healing.

Lord, I want you . . .
    but I don't want you!
Lord, I'm looking for you . . .
    but I can't find you!
Lord, I've deceived myself.
    I thought I wanted your way, but I want mine.
    I thought I wanted your will, but I want mine.
    I thought I wanted your kingdom, but I wanted the world's.

Lord, my life is in conflict.
    Help me to want your way more than I want mine!
    Help me to want your will more than I want mine!
    Help me to want your kingdom more than I want the world's!

Lord, I want your will to be mine
    And your life as an example for mine!

                                        Amen

4 Who Am I?

And Jesus looking upon him loved him, and said to him, "You lack one thing; go, sell what you have, and give to the poor, and you will have treasure in heaven; and come, follow me."

Mark 10:21

ONCE WE HAVE BEGUN TO TURN our wills and our lives over to God, we are in a position to take a more honest and objective look at ourselves. In order to bring about spiritual recovery we need to get in touch with the desires, attitudes, and behavior that help to determine our illness or our health. That is, we need to know our emotional and spiritual assets and liabilities.

Making a realistic assessment of ourselves is a difficult and painful process. Most of us are good at analyzing another person and prescribing what is necessary for that person's health and happiness. But when it comes to ourselves, we are often either blind or cowardly.

Every personality trait can become either an asset or a liability—it can either be used for health or illness. For example, I used to take pride in my ability to be forgiving and understanding. Unfortunately, that also had its negative side, because there were times when I would be so

43

forgiving and understanding that I let people walk on me. Then my "good" trait became a character defect because I was being a martyr unnecessarily. The result of this was feeling hurt, and also being angry at the person who took advantage of me. Of course, I was also angry at myself, because no one could take advantage of me unless I let them.

This resentment was a liability for me. It always came out in destructive behavior. I would get depressed and isolate myself. Or I would compulsively eat or overwork. But one of the most destructive ways that my resentment came out was through my many automobile accidents. One of the most humiliating discoveries I ever made about myself was the awareness that prior to almost every accident I had, I was either angry at myself or someone else. Not only was my resentment unhealthy for me, but for others as well. Fortunately, I didn't kill myself or anyone else.

This was difficult for me to realize. I didn't want to accept the fact that my misdirected anger was the cause of some people, including myself, being physically hurt. But I am not the only one whose misdirected anger could result in self-destructive behavior. Others have this problem, too. We need to be aware of those qualities within ourselves so that we can know when and how they become destructive. This will help us to transform our character traits from weaknesses into strengths. At the same time, we need to remember that we are fallible human beings who are striving to improve, but who will never reach perfection in this life.

Becoming aware of ourselves can be a very distressing process. You might find yourself becoming afraid, resentful, guilty, or depressed. You may find yourself wanting to procrastinate. But do not let yourself do it. And remember, your journey toward self-awareness is not a one-time task.

It is a way of life based on the courage to be honest with ourselves. Unless this is a daily process and unless we allow God to help make it happen, the gifts that God has given us will become liabilities and spiritual recovery will never take place.

To help you gain awareness of yourself, I suggest that you evaluate yourself by using the following character traits. This is a list of personal liabilities and assets used by persons in search of self-knowledge. I would also suggest that you find a quiet place where you could use this list to reflect on your strengths and weaknesses. This will help you to identify them and start you on the way to a more positive life-style.

LIABILITY	ASSET
Fear	Faith
Resentment	Love
Guilt	Forgiveness
Self-pity	Self-respect
Selfishness	Understanding
Phoniness	Responsibility
Dishonesty	Honesty
False pride	Humility
Hypercriticism	Thankfulness
Impatience	Patience
Procrastination	Promptness
Rationalization	Reason

As you study this list, ask God to show you how some of your character traits become liabilities instead of assets.

• Do not rationalize.

• Admit the real reason for your difficulty no matter how distasteful it may be.

- Do not attempt to justify inappropriate or destructive behavior.

- Do not confuse bad temper with righteous indignation.

- Do not confuse stubbornness with determination.

- Do not allow your selfish pride to become "the right" to which you are entitled.

- Do not justify your faulty relationships with others by thinking that you have a right to your own opinion.

- Be open to the spirit of God.

The rich young ruler

Facing ourselves with all our strengths and weaknesses can be a very frightening experience. It is frightening to see our strengths because then we have to stop excusing our inappropriate behavior. It is also hard to look at our weaknesses because then we have to stop trying to make someone else responsible for our destructive behavior. When we see ourselves as we really are we find it painful and are often reluctant to act on what we have discovered.

The rich young ruler (Mark 10:17-22) is an example of this. He had kept all the commandments. He was a successful man. But his values were all mixed up. He had to face the reality that his goals for life were wealth and power, yet this had left his life empty.

When he came to Jesus he was willing to accept responsibility for his life. He asked Jesus what to do. Unlike many who come for help, he was not blaming others, his childhood, or his unhappy surroundings. He was willing to do something—almost anything—to find a more satisfying life.

Jesus helped the rich young ruler reexamine his values. I know many professionals who make the mistake in working with people of not insisting that they look at their value system. Consequently, they can do little to help people because happiness is never found in money, success, or power. Rather, it is found in living in a relationship with God and other people. The rich young man had kept the law, but it seemed as though he had loved *things* more than God and people. He had been grabbing more of everything than he needed, fearing he would not have enough. His life, therefore, was empty and meaningless.

I recall the successful executive and his wife who came to me for marriage counseling. Bob's goal was to become president of his company and to acquire all of the things necessary to make him and his wife happy. But all Bob's wife and children wanted was for him to be a husband and a father. When the promotion did not come, he became despondent and developed a drinking problem. The more he drank the more depressed he became. Finally, his wife felt that things had gone too far. She told him that either he had to change or she was going to leave.

When Bob came to me for counseling, he was desperate. He knew he had to seek help in order to keep his wife and family. But he came for the wrong reason. Most people seek help for the wrong reason. He was going to change so he could control his wife. Ironically, he had grown up in a broken home and had vowed that he was going to be a family man—only to repeat exactly what had happened in his childhood. He gave his family all kinds of things—

ski vacations, Hawaii, an expensive home—but he had not given them himself.

In my work with Bob, I tried to help him see that he was not concerned about changing his own life. I told him that as long as he was only trying to remain in control of his wife, he was wasting his time. Unfortunately, he was unwilling to hear what I was saying and he gave his wife no alternative. When she filed for divorce, Bob's life was shattered. Not only had he lost his dearest possession (he had used people and loved things), but he had created the very situation he had told himself he would avoid—a broken home.

About a year after the divorce, I heard that Bob had died following open heart surgery. In his trauma he had added to his already excessive daily stresses. An organization for people who have had open heart surgery has as its symbol a red heart with a line through it. This implies a broken heart that has been mended. Thus, the group is called Mended Hearts. I am convinced that Bob's death was really more from a broken than a defective heart. Unfortunately, Bob's heart never mended physically or spiritually. Even after surgery he had continued to drive himself toward success and to try to control others, but there was no peace in his life. He never found that peace and serenity which only God's love, grace, and forgiveness can give, because he was unwilling to accept his need for change.

Changed by love

If anything would change the rich young ruler it would be what Jesus did. "Jesus, looking upon him, loved him."

Through this example Jesus taught us that people are motivated to change by someone loving them.

But not always. Bob was loved by his family, by me, and most of all by God. But being loved was too threatening for Bob.

If he had accepted love from others, he would have had to return it, and he had never learned how. For Bob, loving was performing deeds and buying things. It was acting rather than being in relationship with people.

I remember the day Bob's wife told him that she had never wanted all of the things he had acquired. She would have been happy with a shack, if they could share their love. She was loving him and challenging him to change his values. In the same way, Jesus loved the rich young man and told him to "go, sell what you have, and give it to the poor . . . and come, follow me." But Bob's pride and fear of change immobilized him. His pride was saying: "It's not your problem, it's theirs . . ." and his fear was saying: "I'm too nervous to face myself and too weak to change what I don't like."

Not only are we paralyzed by our pride, but sometimes by our fear, as well. However, if we will allow God's love to penetrate our defenses we will find the strength to see that there is meaning in life, and God will help us find what we need to fulfill our life—so that our life will be more positive, constructive, and healthy.

Many factors prevent us from being open to our Lord so that we can look at ourselves. There is the urge not to let go of sinful behavior. The problem with many of us is that one minute we want to give it up and next we want to keep it. We need to ask God to show us how our resentment, pain, or greed binds us and does not allow us to be what God has created us to be.

There is also our false sense of happiness. This, too, gets in the way of looking at ourselves honestly. We have deceived ourselves and we think we are happy doing destructive things. There are many who think that being self-centered gives them happiness. After all, don't they get what they want when they want it? So why give that up—why change it?

Another difficulty is that we try to excuse some of our inappropriate behavior by all the service we do for the church, for our families, or for our neighbors. We sometimes hide behind this in order to avoid the kind of self-analysis we need so that we can give *ourselves* to our Lord. He wants *us*, not the services we perform.

There is the problem too of the person who uses his intellect to escape looking at himself. There are all kinds of people who use the excuse that they do not understand some aspect of religion or life. They think this allows them to avoid any introspection. It is interesting to see how these people operate, because you can help them answer one question and before you know it they have another. Finally, you realize that the problem is not that they do not understand, but that they are either selfish or self-indulgent and do not want to change.

I remember a woman whose life was in shambles. Her husband was an alcoholic, her son was on drugs, and she was just existing. Over a period of about eighteen months of introspection, private therapy and participating in a group, she began to experience God's love. She then began to see what was destructive in her life and what she needed to change.

Interestingly, she found that when she changed, her husband and son also began to change. However, it should be remembered that there is no guarantee that others will change if you do.

Just as this woman began to use her personality, gifts, and love to change herself and help her husband and son, so Jesus told the rich young man to use his talents to enrich the lives of others, rather than accumulate more riches.

The Christian faith has always said that God plays an active part in our life, if we will only be open to his love. And God's wish for us is not that we spend our life acting and reacting, but being the person he created us to be, and living in relationship with him and others so that we can use the gifts he has given us.

The most important thing about change is that God understands how difficult it is. He is aware of the importance of the comfort, support, and encouragement of others around us. He suggested that the rich young man throw in his lot with the rest of the disciples. Jesus wanted the young man to have some personal support in his struggle to change his self-centered life-style. This is why the church is so important and why AA-Alanon-Alateen, Mended Hearts, Emotions Anonymous. Overeaters Anonymous, Oncology Share and Care Groups, and other self-help groups are so important. When we accept God's love and his challenge to become aware of ourselves and change, we need support. We need a fellowship that will hold our hand when we feel alone and be there to pick us up when we stumble and fall. But before that will happen we need to take a moral inventory of ourselves.

I can imagine the rich young ruler contemplating the words of Jesus: "Go, sell . . . , and give to the poor, . . . and come, follow me." As he begins to walk away, you can see that his eyes are focused on the ground. You notice that he is stooped from sadness and that he walks with a slow and aimless gait. You can see the tears in his eyes. Jesus has caused him to look at himself. He is saddened by what he sees. Not only is he going to have to give up his wealth, but he also must change his values.

As he thinks back on that experience with Jesus, he recalls how easily he evaded the challenge of Jesus. He had shut the door on Jesus' love because his selfishness and pride had gotten in the way. Now he was seeing the face of Jesus again in his mind. Two things about Jesus kept coming back to him: that Jesus loved him more than anyone had loved him before, and that Jesus told him what he had to do to find happiness and an abundant life. Jesus believed in him even though he knew the worst about him, and helped him to see what was hindering his spiritual recovery. But I can also imagine the rich young ruler wanting to let go of that which is destructive in his life. For him, possessions had become more important than God and people. I can see him finding the strength from Jesus to overcome his fears of the past, present, and future, and to face himself. I can see him finding the courage to respond to the voice that said: "Come, follow me." And I can see that young man walking through the gates into the new world that Christ offered—the world of power, joy, serenity, and love. It contained sacrifice, but it contained Jesus as well. In the same way, today, Jesus calls to us to face ourselves so that we too might experience a life of power, joy, serenity, and love.

Lord, who am I?

I am at the same time strong and weak,
   forgiving and unforgiving,
   loving and unloving,
   decisive and indecisive,

trusting and distrusting,
rational and irrational,
responsible and irresponsible,
patient and impatient,
feeling and unfeeling.

I am all of these things, Lord, and more . . .
I'm human.

But sometimes I'm more weak than strong . . .
And my life becomes destructive to myself and others.
I let the secondary values of acquiring things and power
take over . . .
I lose sight of you and those important people in my life.

Forgive me, Lord . . .
Help me to see my strengths and my weaknesses
So that I can turn my weaknesses into strengths . . .
So that I can find my strength in my weakness . . .
Because I have turned my will and my life over to you.
Amen

5 Lord, I Confess

Therefore, confess your sins to one another, and pray for one another, that you may be healed. The prayer of a righteous man has great power in its effect.
                                                                    James 5:16

LIVING ALONE WITH OUR PROBLEMS, defects, or sins is one of the most destructive things we can do. These conflicts will plague us, threaten us, and inhibit us often in ways of which we are not even aware. They will control us because we tend to nurse them, expand them, and blow them out of proportion. Admitting to God and to ourselves those thoughts and behaviors that bother us often is not enough, although it is a start. But in addition, we need to talk to some other trusted person.

This step, however, is extremely difficult. It is one thing to admit my faults to God and myself, but it is a totally different thing to admit them to another person. Many of us would rather suffer alone in silence than to confess our sins to someone else.

The practice of confessing our faults to another person is an ancient one. It was common in biblical times, and it has continued to the present time. It is not only a valuable principle in religious life, but it is now encouraged by psychiatrists, physicians, psychologists, social workers, and other health care professionals. It is also the basis of most self-help groups like Alcoholics Anonymous.

Unresolved guilt can be one of the most powerful forces we have in life. It can motivate us to change that which is destructive in our lives, or it can prevent us from being what God created us to be. Guilt is constructive in our lives only when we use it to change that which we don't like about ourselves.

There are two kinds of guilt: real and neurotic. We feel real guilt when we go against our moral value system. This guilt has a rational basis. Neurotic guilt is feeling guilty when we shouldn't. It is irrational. Children sometimes feel responsible for their parents' divorce, or feel that they fall short of the expectations of their parents. Hence they feel false or neurotic guilt. People who seem to feel guilty and apologetic about almost everything they do probably are suffering from neurotic guilt.

There are some persons in our society who feel that guilt has no value at all. This is hard for me to understand, because there are times when we should all feel guilty. People who never experience guilt are either psychopathically ill or cease to be human. They lack a conscience and will probably end up outside the law; or they may abuse others to satisfy their own needs.

Guilt can become a destructive force in our lives when we repress our feelings rather than deal with them constructively. Some people actually choose guilty feelings instead of good feelings. They may do this out of habit, or because it gives them an excuse for not changing their lives—after all, they are too helpless to change; because they get attention (pity) as a result of their hopeless condition; or because they can get others to take responsibility for them. Unfortunately, this can result in people becoming sick—physically, emotionally, and spiritually.

The solution to the illness caused by guilt is forgiveness. However, appropriating God's forgiveness is difficult. Often we need to make confession not only to God and ourselves, but to another person in order to begin the process of accepting God's forgiveness. We need to be forgiven in the name of Jesus Christ, by a professing Christian, as we see in Matthew 18:18 and 19: "Truly, I say to you, whatever you bind on earth shall be bound in heaven, and whatever you loose on earth shall be loosed in heaven. . . . I say to you, if two of you agree on earth about anything they ask, it will be done for them by my Father in heaven." Forgiving another person in the name of Christ is not only a responsibility that we have as Christians, but it is also an opportunity. Being forgiven by another Christian is an added bonus the confessing Christian has going for him, if he will take advantage of it.

The healing of the paralytic

The story of the young man with the paralyzed legs is a good illustration of how the destructive power of guilt can affect a person's physical health. This connection between the body, mind, and spirit was discussed by the ancient Hebrew writers. Jesus knew that sin and health are related and that there is a relationship between a healthy mind and a healthy body. This is why he saw the man's need as basically religious—primarily the assurance of forgiveness.

The paralytic had apparently not handled his guilt feelings appropriately. He had bottled them up. He needed to hear that his sins were forgiven. He needed to confess them to someone else. Jesus took the moral problem seriously. So often Christian counselors or pastors get so caught up with the new psychological fads that they neglect the obvious—that being human is being moral and often the problem is strictly spiritual.

In the case of the paralytic, his unresolved moral conflict had resulted in feelings of guilt and this had led to his becoming physically ill. The turning point was when Jesus told him that his sins were forgiven. Immediately, the young man was able to get up and walk.

I recall working with a teenage girl who was brought into our hospital following an accident. I remember how angry and rebellious she was while she was recovering. During her recovery she gradually lost the use of her legs, even though the accident had not affected them in any way. She had become paralyzed by her feelings. Her anger at her parents and her guilty feelings about that anger had resulted in a temporary paralysis.

The doctors had decided to give her a placebo by injection. She was told this injection could cure her paralysis. This failed. When she was able to resolve her anger and guilt and forgive her parents for "failing" her (there was some question whether they had), she was able to forgive herself, and the paralysis left her.

When we are aware of such situations occurring in our age, it helps us to understand the account of Jesus healing the young paralytic brought to him by four friends. Mark's version uses the term "my son," which would indicate that perhaps this was an adolescent who was caught up in the moral conflict that is common to that stage in life. Perhaps he felt as though he was not living up to his own standards. It is possible that he was having the same kind of difficulty as the young woman who had the accident. He may have been struggling with his own independence or with some questions about the meaning of life, and how frustrating it was not to be able to find his life's purpose.

At any rate, Jesus approached the paralytic with the assumption that he had a spiritual problem. Jesus was not concerned with the symptoms, but with the young man's attitude toward life as a whole. The paralytic's problem was his sense of sin and his need to receive from Jesus the assurance of God's forgiveness. Only when he accepted the unconditional love and forgiveness of God was he healed of his paralyzed state. I am also convinced, even though there is no evidence of this, that this young man confessed his sins to Jesus. Otherwise, I do not believe that he could have accepted God's forgiveness, nor would Jesus have said: "Your sins are forgiven." In other words, the most important thing that the paralytic did was to confess his sin to Jesus. He had not even come to Jesus on his own accord. He had come because of the faith of his four friends, but he had taken advantage of the opportunity—he had opened himself up to God's forgiveness through confession.

The value of confession

There are many people both inside and outside the church who intellectually know God's love revealed in Christ, but who have never experienced it in their hearts. They have never known the fellowship that occurs when they see each other as sinners as well as people of faith. So often we think that we dare not be sinners. We can be sick, but we can't be sinners. To use the word "sin" in our day is forbidden. But God's grace allows us to be sinners.

God wants us to come to him as we are and give him our hearts. But unless we confess our sins to him, to ourselves, and, most important, to another person, we will experience neither the fellowship of other Christians nor the assurance of forgiveness. Rather, we will keep ourselves alone and isolated. And whoever is alone in sin is utterly alone.

Christ gives each of us who claim him as Lord the authority and the opportunity to hear the confession of sin and to forgive sin in his name. He tells us in John 20:23, "If you forgive the sins of any, they are forgiven; if you retain the sins of any, they are retained." When Christ says that, he allows us to share our sin with our brothers and sisters and they can do the same with us. Through confession and the authority to forgive sin in his name, he gives us the power to break out of our tortured loneliness into a fellowship of belonging.

In confession we break out of loneliness and have an opportunity for fellowship and belonging. Sin often forces us to remain by ourselves. In fact, one of the results of sin is separation—separation from God and man. Confession, however, is no guarantee that you will feel that you belong. Confession only gives you the freedom to reach out for fellowship. Belonging takes an effort and a risk, but I hope that after confession you will have the confidence (as a result of beginning the process of forgiveness) to reach out to others and accept the friendship and support of others.

One of the most significant advantages of confession in the presence of another is that it breaks our desire for self-justification. In confession we not only humble ourselves before another person, but we stop excusing our sin. When we admit our wrongs to God, ourselves, and another person, our sin is out in the open. We have given it up.

We are no longer hanging on to it or hiding it. We have given our heart to God. We have been forgiven and reconciled to Christ and our neighbor. Our sin no longer has control over us.

In the confession of our sin to another person, we are also able to give up our false sense of pride. Prior to our confession, we were attempting to be our own God. Confession in the presence of a Christian makes us humble. In the confession of specific sins our false pride dies, and a new pride based on honesty and integrity is born. This is both a painful and a liberating process. Some call it rebirth or being born again.

I remember the Easter Sunday morning several years ago when I decided to speak of my resurrection experience from the pulpit. It was the story of my attempted suicide and resulting discovery of God's forgiving love. I recall how frightening and humiliating it was. But I will also never forget how exhilarated I felt to finally get it out. To tell hundreds of people was like letting the whole world know. For the first time, I felt the joy and the freedom of not having to hide that part of me which I despised the most. I had nothing to be afraid of any more, because everyone knew it. I had finally *let go* of the sin that was controlling my life. I had confessed it to the whole Christian community and to God.

Most of the congregation was loving and forgiving. But the following week I received two unsigned letters telling me how I had "let them down." Apparently, I had been on a pedestal and for the first time they had seen me as a human being and as a sinner. Perhaps my confession of sin was too threatening, because it forced them to get in touch with their own need of confession.

The humiliation of confession is painful, but it is liberating. It allows us to experience God's forgiveness through his act in Christ on the cross. In confessing our sins to our brother/sister in Christ, we experience the rescue, redemption, and resurrection made possible through the cross of Christ.

Confession also allows us to begin a new life. The sins of resentment, false pride, and guilt have been forgiven. There is a break with the sins of the past. Christ has given us a new beginning as we see in 2 Corinthians 5:17: "If anyone is in Christ, he is a new creation; the old has passed away, behold, the new has come." Without confession we are more likely to repeat the same old sins of the past. One of the reasons that some people avoid confession is because they want to continue the things they were doing—they don't want to give up their destructive, sinful ways. Through confession it becomes more difficult to repeat our destructive behavior. Instead, we have a chance to begin a new life because we have broken with the past.

In confession, we find a new sense of certainty about life. By confessing our sins to another Christian, we are able to break the cycle of self-deception and come out of that experience with the assurance of God's forgiveness for *particular* sins. This is possible because we have made confession of specific sins as a result of our self-examination.

In spite of how important confession to another person is, however, it is not a divine law. Martin Luther said in the Small Catechism that the sins we should confess are the sins that bother us. If we have experienced forgiveness without confession to another person and have not deceived ourselves, confession to someone else is not necessary. The important thing is that we be honest with ourselves and share the realization that we are sinners. Not to do that would separate us from the Christian fellowship.

Two important aspects of making a confession are to whom should we confess and why? First, the one we choose as our confessor must be someone who has the wisdom, understanding, and mercy to hear our confession. This person must know the love and forgiveness of God and be able to communicate that to us.

Second, we must keep in mind that our purpose for confession is to experience the forgiveness of sins, not to feel a false sense of pride in our confessing. Confession is a sacred act and to make it less than that means that our pride has gotten in the way and we try once again to be our own God. In confession, we need to make sure that the purpose and goal is the forgiveness of sins.

The confession of our faults to another person who will forgive us in the name of Christ can be one of the most liberating and healing experiences in our lives. In fact, without it, God's forgiving and healing power will not be released in us. For unless we admit to being sinners, we will never admit to needing God.

> Lord, confession is so painful.
> Letting go is so frightening.
> Lord, it's humiliating!
>
> I can't stand it alone!
> Being alone in my sin is being so totally alone!
>
> Keeping it inside is so destructive.
> It's so hard to keep justifying,
>   blaming others,
>   and playing God.
>
> Lord, help me to risk it . . .
>   to open up,
>   to let go,
>   to let you take over.

Lord, help me to trust
  my brothers and sisters in Christ.
Help me to dare to be a sinner,
  to dare to be human . . .
So that I might know
  the joy of confession,
  the liberation of telling another person,
  the support of the fellowship,
  and the exhilaration of being resurrected!

6 Letting Go

> If anyone says, "I love God," and hates his brother, he is a liar; for he who does not love his brother whom he has seen, cannot love God whom he has not seen. And this commandment we have from him, that he who loves God should love his brother also.   1 John 4:20-21

ETTING GO OF OUR DESTRUCTIVE character traits so that God can remove them is very difficult. When a person has been living with a particular life-style it is easier to retain it than to give it up to God. It is familiar and predictable, and gives us an unholy "comfort."

I recall how difficult it was for me to give up my suicidal tendencies. Not only did I overtly attempt suicide, but I covertly continued my destructive ways even after I began to know the love of God. Destructive character traits take time to change. I did not acquire them overnight, and I will not get rid of them easily either.

My primary reason for attempting suicide was that I had turned my anger in on myself and had become depressed. I had isolated myself from people. But I was not so depressed that I could not function. In order to commit suicide, you need enough energy and motivation to act on the anger you have internalized.

After I began my recovery process, I continued to bottle up my anger. I refused to tell people what I thought and felt. Evidence of this was my tendency toward having automobile accidents, as mentioned earlier. Also, I would get depressed from time to time as a lot of people do. Sometimes all my anger would be focused on one event. I remember the day I was trying to get my lawn mower started. I became so furious at its lack of cooperation that I was about to carry it across the street and throw it into the valley. In the process of doing this I began to realize how inappropriate my anger was for the situation. I realized that I was not only angry at the lawn mower, but at a lot of things that had been accumulating for months. My difficulty was that I was storing up the anger and nursing it. The lawn mower episode was the situation which gave me permission in my own mind to let it out.

I had gotten my anger out, but it was still a destructive part of my life. I had to turn it over to God. I had to let him help me with it. I was not certain how I was going to do this, but I knew I had to do it.

At this time I learned the importance of Christian fellowship. Other people had always been there to help, but I had not reached out before. I had prided myself on being able to handle things alone. I had to come to realize that it was okay to be weak at times and allow others to help me. No one can be strong all of the time.

In the process of letting go of my false pride, I found help in a Christian fellowship group. I had come to realize that part of my problem with anger was that I had not learned to tell people when I was angry. Therefore I was turning this anger in on myself. I was resenting myself for allowing others to walk on me. Not only was I being hurt by others, but I was also hurting myself. I detested my behavior which gave others permission to discount me.

By turning my anger over to God and the Christian fellowship, I discovered that I needed to tell people my feelings—especially the negative ones—so I could stop being angry at myself. I had to let go of that behavior so God could give me the strength to change. If my behavior did not change, I would not be able to respect myself. And if I did not learn to like myself I would continue to put myself in a position to be used by others, and the cycle would repeat. I was trapped and I was the only one who could provide the way out of it. I would have to be open to God's strength and to the support of important people in my life; otherwise there would be no possible recovery.

By allowing God to remove our destructive behavior we are beginning to cooperate with him and his will for our lives. God created us for life and not death, for fellowship and not isolation, for health and not illness, and for serenity and not turmoil. This is why he sent us his son. He wanted us to experience the peace, holiness, joy, and community which only he can give—if not fully in this life, then certainly in the life to come.

God did not intend for us to destroy ourselves with alcohol, food, work, stress, or resentment. He created us with the natural inclinations for life, fulfillment, joy, and serenity.

The removal of our destructive character traits requires our cooperation and patience. The problem with many people working on their recovery is their desire to have it happen instantly. We live in an age of instant everything —all the way from instant mashed potatoes to instant headache relief. We need to remember that change takes time.

And we must be *willing* to change. There are a lot of people who try to change or say they will "do the best they can." Unfortunately, this is not enough. I've had people coming to me for months for counseling who are "trying" to change but they are unsuccessful. People often tell me that they are "doing the best they can," but they don't believe there is much they can do. Often this becomes a good excuse for not changing.

We need to desire (more than anything else) to turn our character defects over to God. This is crucial to our recovery. This desire, however, is often aroused when the pain and discomfort of our present situation becomes so great that we are willing to do anything to make it go away.

I recall a depressed middle-aged woman who was not responding to the treatment she was receiving as an outpatient. I recommended that she be put into the hospital and the decision was made to give her electroshock therapy. The purpose of this treatment is to help the patient forget the cause of the depression. After the patient had had two treatments she began to respond very rapidly. When I talked with her about this she told me the reason this was so helpful was actually because she was afraid of having any more treatments. Normally, this is not that threatening for people, but for her the threat of having more treatments motivated her to "want" to do what she had to do to get well. Her present situation was more uncomfortable than the fear she had about changing.

The important thing in letting go is that we commit ourselves to make a beginning, and keep working at it. It is not important how halting we are or how often we fall, but rather how committed we are and how willing we are to let go of those things which we thought we could never live without.

The struggle of Zacchaeus

The story of Zacchaeus as recorded in Luke 19:1-10 illustrates the struggle of one man for power which led to his alienation and separation. Here also is an indication of how a person who is destroying himself was able to be restored to community and serenity.

Zacchaeus is a typical example of modern man. The feeling of isolation is a trademark of contemporary urban life. Thousands of people today are haunted by the feeling of alienation. Sometimes those who have meaningful intimate relationships are insensitive to those who are crying out for fellowship. We assume that most people are just as content as we are. Yet so often the opposite is true —even among those who have supposedly made it in our society.

Most of us have experienced the discomfort of feeling isolated. I remember how alone I felt while teaching in Germany one summer. I was forced to teach in German and barely knew the language well enough to get along. But as the quarter went on I began to get depressed. At mid-term I went on a retreat for a few days near Frankfurt. Then I realized why I was depressed—I felt isolated. Even though I conversed adequately in German, I still felt alone as a result of the language and cultural barriers. At times I am sure I missed out on the full meaning of what was being said because I didn't know the idiomatic expressions people used. I am convinced there were those who thought I was acting "superior" to them because of my hesitant interchanges. My isolation was caused by a communication problem, and it resulted in depression. Prolonged isolation can also cause physical, emotional, and spiritual illnesses.

Being aware of this should help us understand Zacchaeus better. He was excluded from relationships and rejected by his own people. He had chosen to serve the enemy by becoming a tax collector. Therefore, Zacchaeus had been ostracized by his own community.

Those who are familiar with the story of Zacchaeus remember that he was a short man. This was part of the reason why he decided to climb a tree when Jesus came to his city. He wanted to be able to see him. But a more profound reason for climbing the tree was his fear of meeting people face-to-face, and of being involved in any way. There was a very logical reason for his behavior; Zacchaeus was "up a tree" for more than one reason.

When Zacchaeus was found by Jesus, he was telling Jesus by his position in the tree that he wanted help. Significantly, Zacchaeus could have remained "up a tree" and been rejected and despised. But he made the choice to change. No matter how terrifying it was for him to come down and meet Jesus face to face, he decided to do it. He wanted to *let go* of his isolation and the feeling of rejection and let Jesus take charge of his life.

Zacchaeus had made the conscious choice to face life and his own people with the help of Jesus. He was able to do this because he was willing to let go of past resentments toward his own people and the fear of being involved intimately with others. He had found a courage and serenity in Jesus that had enabled him to forgive those who had hurt him and to trust those who had rejected him.

The example of Zacchaeus is important for us because

it shows that people can, if they will, rise above their past. He could change from being a traitor to his own people, from being dishonest and underhanded, from being a Quisling, and turn his life over to God.

Letting Jesus change his life was not easy. Zacchaeus was like most of us who have wanted to change—he found it hard to seek help openly. We sometimes wish something or someone would force us to look for help, so it would be easier to get started. It was almost as if Jesus had created a crisis for Zacchaeus. He pointed him out before the whole crowd. He called him down from the tree, because he wanted to stay at his house that night. Zacchaeus was up against it. If he had refused to come down he would have received even more rejection. He had had all of that he could stand. Besides, here was the man Jesus, whom everyone wanted to know, accepting him in front of all those people. How could he possibly say no?

The change was made possible for Zacchaeus too because he could tell how much Jesus cared for him. After all, Jesus risked accepting Zacchaeus in full view of his enemies. Indeed, Jesus had created a crisis for Zacchaeus by risking himself with a crowd who considered Zacchaeus their enemy. Jesus placed himself in an intimate relationship with Zacchaeus by going to his home. He trusted Zacchaeus enough to allow him to take care of his physical need for food and lodging, as well as his emotional and spiritual need of companionship. In doing this, Jesus accepted him for what he could *become.* Jesus did not merely accept him as he was; he accepted him for what he ought to be. This gave Zacchaeus the courage to become what he was capable of being.

We do not know what they talked about in Zacchaeus' home, but whatever it was, it resulted in a dramatic change. Zacchaeus promised Jesus that he would make reparation for the wrongs he had done. This is the first indication that Zacchaeus had changed. The culmination of this alteration in the life of Zacchaeus, however, was his salvation. When Jesus told him that salvation had come to him he meant that Zacchaeus had been healed. This was possible because he had let go of his past sinful behavior. He had opened himself up to God and to his neighbor and been reconciled to them. Through this reconciliation Zacchaeus had healed his relationships with his own people and with God.

God was able to come into his life because Zacchaeus was willing to do something about his relationship with others. Without a meaningful relationship with our neighbor, we are also out of relationship with God. We need to let go of our wrongs in order to love God. In 1 John 4:20 we read: "If anyone says, 'I love God' and hates his brother he is a liar; for he who does not love his brother whom he has seen, cannot love God whom he has not seen."

Therefore, healing will only occur when we let go of the character defects that destroy our relationships with others, so that we can allow God to accomplish his will in us. We need to "Let go and let God."

Letting go . . .
   of what, Lord?
What do you expect anyway . . .
   Perfection?

I don't know why it's so hard.
I don't know why I hang on so long.
It's so threatening.
I feel so exposed and vulnerable.

My resentment is my courage,
My guilt is my motivation,

My fear is my justification, and
My denial is my strength.

What is there to take its place?
I'm supposed to "let go and let God?"
I have to "let go" so that I can "let God . . ."
  be my courage, motivation, justification, and strength.

Lord, help me to "let go,"
  and keep on letting go!

7 Remove My Shortcomings, Lord

Create in me a clean heart, O God; and put a new and right spirit within me.   Psalm 51:10

AFTER WE HAVE LET GO of our destructive character traits, we may think that we have arrived. We have experienced moments of real peace of mind. We are beginning to experience freedom from guilt, depression, and anxiety. This newfound serenity is a priceless gift.

Prior to letting go of our defects, we were running from pain and trying to avoid problems. We did not want to face the difficult aspects of relationships or the reality of suffering. Most of our energy was used in escaping reality and responsibility.

I remember how good I felt after I let go of my resentment toward my father for not being the father I thought he should have been. I used to blame him for my unwillingness to spend time with him instead of accepting responsibility for my own behavior. When I began to understand why he was not more of a father to me and when I was willing to accept responsibility for my own behavior,

I was able to forgive him and myself as well. When this happened I felt a real sense of peace. I thought I had been relieved of my resentment.

Gradually, I realized that I was also angry at God, because I thought he had let me down. But it was I who had let him down. I realized, too, I was angry at my mother for dying. It was not her fault that she died of cancer when I was seven years old. But I missed her and it hurt to lose her. It was years later that I became aware of my anger at her. So you see, asking God to remove your shortcomings is a lifelong process.

Not only do we continue to find shortcomings that need to be removed, but we are plagued with one vice of which no person in the world is free. It is a weakness we loathe when we see it in others. In fact, most people do not even recognize that they have this shortcoming. I have heard people admit that they have a chemical problem, are bad-tempered, are unfaithful to their spouse, are a "foodaholic," or have problems with depression, anxiety, or fear. But most people are not conscious of this problem. And the more we have this problem in ourselves the more we dislike it in others. The vice I am referring to is false pride. Please notice that I used the term "false pride." It is appropriate to have self-respect, to care for oneself, and to have a *healthy* sense of pride in what we accomplish. But the need to be better than someone else is false pride; and the basis of all of our sins and all our shortcomings is false pride.

The greatest sin

Some may think that I am emphasizing this way out of proportion—that false pride is a problem but it is not the *worst* problem we have. Not only is pride behind most of our sinning—it always results in discontent.

Have you ever wondered why you resent people who snub you or who show off? Because of false pride. False pride is essentially competitive. It desires to be better, or possess more, than the next person. Our false pride takes pleasure in putting someone else down or in seeing others fail. False pride gets no joy out of having something, only out of having more than the next person. This is why it is false. There are some people who are rightly proud of what they have accomplished in life. But the person who is full of false pride feels good only when he is richer, wiser, or better looking than others.

Most of the evils in the world that people blame on greed or selfishness are more likely the results of false pride. Greed will drive a person into competition if there is not enough to go around; but the person who is possessed by false pride will try to get more, just to assert his power. The desire to be richer than others is the wish for power. What gives pleasure to the person with false pride is power. There is nothing that makes a person feel more superior than power. If I am filled with false pride, then anyone who has more power—whether it be in the form of money or wisdom—is my enemy.

False pride has been the primary problem of every individual, family, and nation since the beginning of time. Other vices often bring people together. At times drunken or unchaste people may find companionship with each other. But people who are filled with false pride only find enmity—enmity toward other people and toward God.

Our relationship with God must be based on his superiority. But as long as we are filled with false pride we cannot recognize the superiority of God. Yet we have no trouble convincing ourselves that God approves of us and sees us as being better than others. Whenever our spiritual life results in our feeling that we are better than others we should be aware that our spiritual recovery is being corrupted.

This is why recovery is difficult and why health is so elusive. Many people can correct certain shortcomings in their lives. I have seen many people stop drinking, overcome fear, lust, ill temper, greed, and selfishness, and then become filled with a false sense of power over having done it. They have eliminated the symptom but not the cause of sin.

This does not mean that removing the symptom is not important; it certainly is. Often we cannot work on the cause until the symptom is gone. But we must remember that eliminating the symptom is only the beginning of spiritual recovery. Spiritual recovery means the absence of false pride—it means humility. And the beginning of humility is the realization that we, like most people, are plagued by a false sense of power at times. Unless we accept this we will never experience humility.

Jesus removed the unclean spirits

The account in Mark 5:1-20 of the Gadarene demoniac is the predicament of those who feel possessed by a power outside themselves. This is a phenomenon that is well known in our day. The biblical term for this is demon possession.

I believe there are those who are possessed by a power outside themselves today. But most people are possessed by powers within themselves—resentment, guilt, fear, and denial, to mention a few. Some of these people would like to think they are demon possessed so they can avoid taking responsibility for resolving their problem. There are too many people like this in our society who do not want to face reality and responsibility for their own lives. Unfortunately, there are those who foster this belief by telling people that they have no control over their destiny. These individuals are advocating the idea that people's lives are either predetermined or possessed, and people have neither responsibility nor choice in what happens. To believe this is to deny one's humanity.

The demoniac had been possessed since birth. He had had a war going on inside of him. His conflict had become so intolerable that he was lashing out at the world around him. He was angry at himself and at the feelings he had within of many voices clamoring to be heard. This is why his response to Jesus when asked, "What is your name?" was: "My name is Legion; for we are many" (Mark 5:9).

The way Jesus decides to help him is to restore his dignity as a human being. He saw the illness as a loss of dignity. Jesus saw beneath the angry behavior and realized that his main problem was fear. I have often seen individuals who appear to be very angry, but whose basic problem is fear.

I remember the young couple who came for marriage counseling. After seeing them for some time they determined that they did not want to live together any more because their love had turned to hatred. He was alcoholic and she was from a home where she had never learned to love. Consequently, both of them were afraid of intimacy. He avoided it by drinking and she avoided it by anger. She, of course, felt justified in being this way because of his drinking.

However, she remained an angry person long after the

divorce. So she decided to try to resolve her anger by forgiving those people in her past, including her husband, with whom she had been angry. When she let go of the anger she felt afraid and insecure. She had difficulty functioning because she had never faced her feelings of inadequacy before—she had covered it up with her anger. In addition, she had never had to face the possibility of real intimacy with anyone before because her anger kept people away. The thought of being without her shield of anger was terrifying.

So it was with the demoniac. Jesus knew that his problem was fear. Jesus approached him with patience and understanding and the demoniac calmed down. He could tell that Jesus wasn't afraid of him and most of all that Jesus understood and was able to identify with him.

I remember the woman who had come to our emergency room with her husband who had been accidentally shot and killed. No matter what I did I could not get any response from her. The shock of her husband's death had immobilized her. She was sitting on a couch in the emergency waiting room with her head down, staring at the floor. Finally, I decided to get on my knees, take hold of her hands, and look directly into her eyes. As I did this, she must have realized that I cared, and that I was trying to identify with her. When our eyes met she burst into tears. Shortly she began to speak and she talked of her disbelief, pain, and loss. In the episode with Jesus, the demoniac responded in a similar way. Jesus let him know that he understood and could identify with him.

When Jesus asked him the question: "What is your name?", it was like asking him to tell Jesus about his problem and how it began. Whether or not he and Jesus went into all the causes of his illness, we don't know. But the final scene shows the demoniac restored and sitting talking with Jesus. Jesus had broken through the wall of hostility and isolation to a relationship with him. Jesus had walked with him into the depths of his being to places where he was afraid to walk alone. Through the process of sharing himself with Jesus, he was healed.

Jesus says: "Come out of the man, you unclean spirit." Here Jesus is aware that this man is being controlled by his anger and is driven by fear. He is aware of his potential for good and evil, love and hate, tenderness and rigidity, sensitivity and impatience. Jesus is aware of how much the demoniac wants to change and he is impressed with his humility in that he was willing to admit his need for change. By saying: "Come out of the man," Jesus is letting him know that he understands his anger but that he must not allow it to control his life. He is also letting him know that he can do something about his fear as well, but he has to take responsibility for it.

By encouraging the demoniac to be responsible for helping himself, he is helping to restore his dignity—the dignity that comes from having done something to help himself.

Often we see people who are emotionally ill because of their conflict and struggle to find meaning and direction for their lives. Illness is often the unconscious choice when there seems to be no solution and no hope. Restoring health then is helping them to see that there is a solution, if they are willing to take responsibility for bringing it about, regardless of the pain involved. This will not happen unless we are humble enough to desire God's help and the help of others.

It is no wonder that the demoniac wanted to remain with Jesus. After all, Jesus had loved him enough to help him unscramble his life. He had found meaning for his life and he thought he might lose it if he did not stay with Jesus. But Jesus wanted him to grow in dignity and self-respect, and this would not happen if he remained tied to Jesus. The real test of his recovery was to go back home. Now he was no longer preoccupied by his own conflicts, but filled with the desire and challenge to share what had happened to him and to show the importance of one's relationship to God. He was not thinking only of himself (false pride); he was concentrating on his relationship to God and to his own people because of the wholeness he had found. He was no longer plagued by his self-centered fears, but he had found serenity because he humbled himself and reached out to God and to others.

Healing or spiritual recovery require the absence of false pride—they take humility. Otherwise our reaching out to God will only be halfhearted. We must honestly want him to remove our shortcomings and free us from the powers within and without that control us.

> Lord, remove our shortcomings,
>   but not now, Lord!
> Remove them,
>   but not that one, Lord!
>
> Lord, it's so hard . . .
>   Maybe I've removed
>   fear, lust, greed, impatience, or selfishness . . .
>   Maybe I've let go of my addiction to
>   alcohol, work, food, or procrastination . . .
>
> But are they still present in my life,
>   and in my relationships with others?
> And even worse, Lord, I blow myself up with false pride
>   over the delusion of my superiority to others.

Lord, it's so hard to be humble,
  to remove all my shortcomings,
  never to be conceited,
  never to look down on others.

Lord, help me to look up,
  so I can see you!
For it is in seeing you,
  that I will find humility.

These
8 I Have
Harmed

So if you are offering your gift at the altar, and there remember that your brother has something against you, leave your gift there before the altar and go; first be reconciled to your brother, and then come and offer your gift. Matthew 5:23-24

WHEN I ASKED GOD to remove my shortcomings I was on my way to recovery. And it was a good beginning! But completing the steps to recovery was an ongoing process. Coming to terms with those I have harmed by thought or deed is a vital and important part of recovery—whether physical, emotional, or spiritual. *The New Testament makes it very clear that it is impossible to have a relationship with God if my relationships with people are not right.* And if there is no relationship with God, there will be no serenity.

To make a list of those we have harmed and to become willing to make amends is very difficult. If we have lied to them or cheated them we have probably caused them spiritual and emotional pain. If we have an uncontrolled temper, we may have hurt them physically and emotionally. If our sex life is selfish, we may have caused misery and a desire for retaliation. There are more subtle ways of harming others, too—like being irritable, cold, irresponsible, impatient, grumpy, or domineering. Or we may wallow in depression and self-pity.

Besides making a list of those we have harmed, being willing to make amends, and changing our behavior, we also need to restore broken relationships with people. If we have to apologize and make up for harmful behavior we are less likely to repeat it. This is the concept that Jesus is talking about in Matthew 5:23-24.

Many people want to have God on their side, but they do not want to give up a resentment or grievance. If only they will make a list of those they resent, seek them out if possible, talk things over, forgive them so they can get rid of the malice in their hearts, they will experience joy, peace, and serenity.

Jesus points out that it is not repentance that is essential for forgiveness, but it is our forgiveness of others. In order to claim our forgiveness, we need to forgive those who have injured us or are in our debt. There is no other petition in the Lord's Prayer that has a condition attached to it except the prayer for forgiveness.

In Matthew 18:23-35 Jesus tells the parable of the unforgiving servant. This is the story of a servant who owed his king ten thousand talents. The king ordered him and his family to be sold in order to pay the debt. The servant begged the king to spare him, so the king released him and forgave him the debt. But that servant was unwilling to forgive one of his own servants a small debt and threw him into prison. When the king heard this he summoned his servant to come to him, rebuked him, put him in jail, and told him that he would have to stay there until his debt was paid. "So also my heavenly Father will do to every one of you, if you do not forgive your brother from your heart" (Matthew 18:35).

Jesus is making it very plain that there is no such thing as a private reconciliation with God. Unless our relationships are right with people they are not right with God either and there is no forgiveness. Attempting to recover while refusing to mend relationships with those we have hurt is not only avoiding reality but losing out on the greatest blessing of all—serenity.

Unless we have resolved that aspect of ourselves which has caused us to be separated from others, we will not have peace of mind and we will be separated from God. God is seeking us, but we will not be found if we refuse to forgive our neighbor and make amends.

Health involves making amends

Not only is it important to make amends to those I have harmed to attain emotional health, but it is necessary for physical health as well. Physicians have known for a long time that physical illness can be caused by unresolved resentment, fear, guilt, false pride, sorrow, or other psychic pain. There are many situations in which the physical disorder appears to be an emotional necessity. A person's reaction to being treated for a physical problem may be to develop another illness, more serious than the first. Here the emotional difficulty is converted into a physical disorder.

I remember the Danish student who came here to study, but he found the social life more interesting than the academic. When examination time arrived, he became sick with a stomach problem and had to be sent back home, because his condition did not seem to improve.

This was a real illness, but one from which he recovered easily when he was back home. If we have no apparent way of solving an emotional conflict except by a psychosomatic illness, then we may unconsciously choose that, and be just as sick as if we had appendicitis.

Most of us can cite examples of where we have wanted to "get off the hook" and our body has done it for us. I remember my cases of diarrhea in college when I wanted to get out of something. However, it was usually only a temporary difficulty and although it helped me to avoid things for a while, I eventually had to face the situation anyway.

Not only do people sometimes develop physical illnesses to avoid unpleasant situations, but there is much evidence now that diabetes, for example, can be triggered by an emotional crisis. In a recent study of 25 cases, 20 of them had a recent crisis in their lives—like a loss of someone close to them, or they had suffered a severe personal loss. Their diabetic condition was the result of their trauma.

Most sexual dysfunctions result from emotional conflicts. There are all kinds of situations where a couple thought that one or the other, or both, were sterile. Following the adoption of a child, however, they found they were able to have children of their own.

There are many questions being asked about immunity today. Studies show that stress slows down the formation of antibodies to fight disease. There are many who believe that unresolved stress can affect our resistance to cancer, because stress can interrupt the immune mechanism of the body.

Some studies show that most heart attacks come during sleep and often during dreaming. This suggests that the emotional content of certain dreams may be the stimulus for many heart attacks that occur during the night when the heart is supposed to be resting. Consequently, stress can have a negative effect on the functioning of the heart. Maybe this is one of the reasons that Paul said: "Be angry but do not sin; do not let the sun go down on your anger" (Ephesians 4:26).

I recall a situation that happened with one of our emergency chaplains. He was on duty when a call came to go out with the ambulance. The police had found a 47-year-old man who had just died. They had called for the chaplain because they felt that someone should call on his wife. She told the chaplain that when she left her husband only an hour earlier, he was feeling fine. The chaplain spent a great deal of time with the wife at the hospital, but he left feeling uneasy over how emotionally upset she was. The wife was left in the care of family, neighbors, and her pastor. But one week to the day later the wife died of an apparent stroke in our Intensive Care Unit. She had collapsed at the reviewal and had been brought in by ambulance. I am convinced that the stress resulting from the loss of her husband was what triggered her stroke and subsequent death.

I also remember the woman in our cardiac unit who spoke to her doctor and me about five minutes before she had her cardiac arrest. She told us she wanted to die. She talked of having nothing more to live for because at 61 she was divorced and her ten children were grown. She was not only suffering the grief of losing her husband, but the grief of the "empty nest syndrome." This was the way out of her meaningless life.

The growing process of children can also be interrupted by emotional stress. This is controlled by the secretion of the pituitary gland and it can apparently be suspended by the stress caused by conflict in the home. I am also aware of several situations from family counseling experiences where children at seven or eight developed ulcers or colitis. I remember the seven-year-old who was blaming himself for his parents' separation and developed an ulcer. Whenever children are unsure of their environment, similar consequences may result.

Unresolved conflicts, resentments, and losses can result in painful memories and meaninglessness, and people can consciously or unconsciously choose illness as a way out. This illness, as we have seen, can even result in death. But when people have meaningful lives and are able to resolve their conflicts—whether indecision, resentment or loss— they invariably choose health over illness.

I recall the situation of the woman who was going to have goiter surgery. The day of the operation she was so anxious that the physician did not want to risk the surgery. She went to a psychiatrist to get help for her anxiety and returned to the doctor six months later without the anxiety and without the goiter.

Many situations have occurred where healing has taken place because of one's faith. Not only have people believed in their physician, but most of all in the power of God to heal. There are other situations where a person's tensions, fears, guilts, and griefs have been resolved and the patient has become physically and emotionally well because a spiritual solution to the problem had been found—such as faith, hope, forgiveness, or reconciliation.

The importance of unconscious emotions

One of the most important aspects of identifying those we may have hurt is by trying to recall the hostilities, fears, conflicts, sorrows, guilts, and painful memories of the past. Most people are controlled more by their unconscious thoughts than they are by their conscious thinking. It is estimated that 70% of our behavior is motivated by our unconscious mind. If this is true, then it is apparent that we need to become more aware of ourselves. Otherwise, we will not be able to do anything to resolve those negative attitudes which result in destructive physical reactions.

Conscious knowledge of those feelings that we need to resolve is difficult enough, but when we are not aware of what we are feeling—let alone not having reconciled these feelings—we may need some help in identifying them. Here are some ways of becoming aware of unconscious thoughts:

1. Talking about our feelings with someone we trust
2. Writing about the feelings
3. Recording our dreams
4. Reflecting on our past destructive behavior
5. Meditating and praying

Let me elaborate on these ideas so that you understand what I mean. First, to talk to another person about something which you yourself are not sure of may sound ridiculous, but it works. Maybe sometime you have started to talk to someone and you surprised yourself by coming out with something you had not thought of before, and you said to yourself, "I didn't know I felt that way!" I have often used the statement with people: "I don't know what I think; I haven't said it yet."

When you are feeling upset but do not know exactly

what you are feeling you could start by saying: "I don't know what I'm feeling, but I'm feeling uncomfortable and I want to talk about it." I remember being at a retreat about 8 or 10 years ago and discovering how hurt and angry I was over my mother's death. I had buried this for 25 years because it was too painful to face. (I am sure this has had a lot to do with why I never married. One way to avoid the pain of loss is not to take the chance of losing again.) After discovering the anger I felt toward my mother, I needed to forgive her, even though she was dead, so I could finally let go of it. I think I had been denying that I was angry at her for all those years because a good child does not resent his parents—especially, it was not okay to be angry at someone who had died.

Second, making the effort to write out your thoughts is also a way of being more aware of your feelings. Often people who need to reconcile themselves with one of their parents find that writing a letter to them without mailing it is a helpful method of expressing their feelings—especially the resentment, guilt, fear, and loss—that need healing. You see, our minds tend to repress the things that have hurt us. It is our challenge to become aware of these hurts and stop denying them so that we can make amends.

Most of us find it easier to admit that we have a poorly functioning heart or gland than to admit we are harboring resentment, fear, guilt, or sorrow. If our body is ill or in pain we can plead that we are victims of fate, and there is nothing we can do to prevent it. If it has anything to do with our emotional or spiritual health we feel responsible and may see a need to accept that responsibility to become aware of our unconscious pains and resolve them.

Third, recording our dreams is another way of getting in touch with our unconscious emotions. If we have a disturbing dream we need to get up, even if it is in the middle of the night, and write it down so that we do not forget it. If we wait until morning we will probably be unable to remember it.

I recall the young boy who was continually having dreams about being eaten by a monster. When he and I talked about what this dream meant to him he spoke about his feelings of insecurity, of not measuring up to his older brother, his health problem, and his fear of losing one or both of his parents because of their marriage difficulty. The boy's ultimate fear was of his own death, just as the basis of all fear, for most of us, is the fear of death. After several counseling sessions, when he began to feel more worthwhile as a person and he was assured that his parents were not going to get a divorce, his nightmares disappeared. Fortunately, it was through his dreams that his parents became aware of his problem.

The fourth way to become more aware of our unconscious thoughts is to reflect on our past destructive behavior. One of the best ways to change bad behavior is to understand why it occurs. Often the real reasons are hidden. For example, I discovered that my tendency to be accident-prone was due to not handling my anger constructively. I would never have known that my unconscious, unresolved anger was the cause, if I had not taken the time to examine what my behavior was "saying." And I probably would have continued the denial process had not my behavior caused me so much pain. Without the pain and the willingness to look at what caused the pain, I would not have known that I needed to resolve my harmful thoughts in order to prevent my destructive behavior from continuing.

Finally, meditation and prayer can make us more aware

of our unconscious mind. The problem with most of us today is that we are too busy, often with insignificant things. We are so busy "running" that we are not *being*. And the only way we can *be* is to be aware of who we are. This can be helped if we will learn to spend some time alone with ourselves and with God in meditation and prayer. In this relationship to God, many people have found a way of discovering those painful memories which tend to be destructive to them physically, emotionally, and spiritually, and God has given them the courage to face them. A beautiful illustration of this is the Psalmist who, in his conversation with God, finds the places within himself which need to be healed and uses his time with God to get his will in tune with God's will so that he can allow God to heal him.

These are some of the methods that may help us to recognize those we have harmed by thought, word, or deed. These are the people with whom we need to make amends. Becoming aware of these conscious and unconscious memories that need healing is necessary to maintain our health. In fact, unless we discover these painful memories which are often unconscious, we not only separate ourselves from God and our neighbors but we increase the possibility of our becoming physically, emotionally, and spiritually ill.

Lord, making a list of those I have harmed is hard enough,
    but discovering the secret thoughts and desires
    which I do not fully know or understand . . .
    is even harder.

I know now, Lord, how important that is.
I know the despair that can come from
    unresolved resentment, guilt, and fear.
I know how loneliness, sorrow, and ambivalence
    can even result in
        illnesses of the body, mind, and soul.

Lord, give me the strength to persevere,
   to be rational,
   to be reflective, and
   to be open to God's will.

Grant me this, Lord,
   so that I might admit my harmful thoughts and deeds . . .
Not only the conscious
   but especially the unconscious.
So I might forgive the wrongs done to me,
   both the real and the imaginary.

Lord, furnish me with an objective view
   so that I will not be too harsh on myself or others,
      nor magnify others' defects or my own.
Lord, give me the desire to mend
   and to make amends.

                                        Amen

Help
9 Me Make
Amends

So whatever you wish that men would do to you,
do so to them; for this is the law and the proph-
ets.   Matthew 7:12

WE ARE NOW READY TO WORK on an appropriate
attitude and making amends wherever possible. We must by this time have made a list
of those we have wronged. We must be more
aware of the unconscious pain needing to be resolved.
Also, we must have faced the reality that we would rather
continue to deny our pain than to begin moving toward
recovery.

Those individuals with whom we need to be reconciled
take on different degrees of importance. Those who are
most important in our lives will obviously be primary.
They will be people like our spouses, parents, children,
and siblings. There will be others that we have harmed
who are not any less significant as far as obtaining our
serenity, such as relatives, friends, neighbors, and other
acquaintances. There will also be those that we will be
unable to contact either because they are deceased, or
because we do not know where they are. There will be

others where efforts toward reconciliation are better left undone because it may result in more injury than healing.

Don't blow it!

The key to making amends is not only to be willing, but to have a loving and forgiving attitude. We can have the best intentions in the world, be willing to talk to all the people we have harmed and still "blow it," because we have not approached these people with an attitude of reconciliation and a desire for restitution. Scripture tells us that one of the signs of Christian maturity is whether or not we are "speaking the truth in love" (Ephesians 4:15). If we are dishonest the relationship has no integrity, and if we are hateful the relationship has been badly ruptured or completely severed. This is why it is so important to know why we want to make amends. Is it to put him in his place? Is it to put her down? Is it to show them how much they have hurt us? Is it to show them how good we are because we are confessing our faults? Or is it to make amends so that we can restore relationships?

I remember the man who had gone through treatment for alcoholism but had become bogged down in his recovery. He came to me for help, and after a short time it was obvious that his trouble was originating from his relationship to his father whom he had not forgiven. I told him that unless he was willing to do this he would not have any peace of mind and, worse than that, he would probably start drinking again.

He saw the truth in that, and agreed to talk to his father. But instead of going to his father with a forgiving attitude, he went intending to tell him just how much he had hurt him and more specifically how he had ruined his life. Naturally, when he left his father, the man was feeling much worse than he did before he came. Not only was he still angry at his father, but now he felt guilty about the way he handled his feelings. He still "needed" the resentment he felt toward his father, because he was not ready to accept the responsibility for his own life.

This is one of the major reasons why many want to hang on to their resentment. Like this man, they don't want to be responsible for their own lives. This attempt at making amends turned out to be nothing more than getting even. The man should not have gone to his father until he had forgiven him in his heart. The only way that we will not blow our experience of making amends is to begin the reconciliation in our hearts before we attempt to make direct amends with those we have harmed.

There are other times when we blow it because we do not think an evil thought is as bad as an evil deed. Admittedly, there are many evil thoughts that do not result in any deed or overt act. But our Lord reminds us in the Sermon on the Mount that the thought is as destructive as the deed, because the thought precedes the deed and it results in separation, and separation is sin (Matthew 5:27f.). Often we may think that there is nothing in regard to our evil thoughts about which we need to make amends. But there is!

Unfortunately, our destructive feelings come out one way or another. We may not have said or done anything that hurt people, but we may have hurt them more by our silence and our avoidance of any relationship at all. Denying our need to resolve our negative feelings, whether they resulted in hurtful behavior or not, will result in our blowing it because we have not given ourselves the right to peace of mind.

There is still one other way in which we could make a mess of making amends. We need to have a sense of self-forgiveness. This should be a part of our experience because of our willingness to make amends with those we have injured. Knowing that we are willing to do what we can to mend relationships should help us feel good enough about ourselves to begin to accept God's forgiveness. Unless we have begun the process of forgiving ourselves, we will not have the courage and perseverance from God to make restitution. Certainly, the process of forgiving ourselves will not be completed until we have forgiven and made direct amends with those we have wronged. Resolving the alienation in our lives takes action, but it begins with a feeling of well-being and forgiven-ness.

Making direct amends

In the case of Zacchaeus, referred to in Chapter 6, Jesus did not tell him that he had to make amends, but he knew that unless he did he would not be able to mend the relationship that he had broken, nor would he be right with God. Zacchaeus began making restitution by making right whatever wrongs he could. "If I have defrauded anyone of anything, I will restore it fourfold" (Luke 19:8).

Often it is not as easy for us as it was for Zacchaeus. Paying back money is not hard if we have it. It is not even hard many times to know what we need to do to resolve the alienation we have helped to create. The hardest thing is doing what we need to do. So often our false pride gets in the way of doing what we know is right.

Part of this hesitation is also due to our knowing that

100

not every attempt to put things right will be met with tears of joy and our being embraced. Sometimes we will be met with contempt, silence, and indifference. I am convinced though that the negative responses will be minimal and the payoffs great. In fact, making direct amends is often the behavior that changes people's lives.

I met a man in the office once who came to me because he was chronically depressed. His wife told him that she couldn't handle it any more. Either he went for help or she was going to leave him. This may sound drastic, but then most of us don't get help unless we are forced into it. After a few sessions it was apparent that his resentment of his domineering mother was one of the paralyzing elements in his life. I told him that he was going to have to forgive her; otherwise he would never be able to take charge of his life. I also told him that he would have to forgive before he talked to her, otherwise he would blow it.

The day came when he went to visit his mother. She didn't fully understand what he was talking about, but there was a reconciliation that occurred between himself and his mother. When he forgave his mother, he was able to break with the past. In the past, he had learned a destructive life-style. His mother did not allow him to express his anger, so he repressed it and became depressed. At times he would become so depressed that he would go to bed and stay there for days. This was not only the way he handled his depression, but it was also his way of punishing his mother—now she had to take care of him. This behavior had continued into his marriage. Now he was punishing his wife and family—most of the time for things they did not do. It was his way of coping with anger.

Since that day of reconciliation, I have not heard that

he has ever become so depressed that he has stayed in bed. Through some additional help he learned to short-circuit his depression by dealing with anger appropriately. When he was not able to prevent his depression, he would not allow himself to go to bed until he had talked it out. Going to bed did not help solve the problem. He was learning to make amends. This had changed his life from being powerless over his depression to being able to be in charge of it and to cope with it.

Making direct amends may mean apologizing to those we have offended, hoping that they will forgive us. Their forgiveness is not necessary if we hope to mend the relationship. The only forgiveness that any of us needs is God's. We are told that we have this because of what Christ has done for us on the cross. All we need to do is confess our sins (1 John 1:9). However, we will have difficulty forgiving ourselves if we do not feel we deserve it. The only way that we will feel assured of this is if we have made amends and changed our hurtful style of living.

Mending relationships may mean making every effort to repair the damage we have done. It may mean confessing jealous, bitter, or envious thoughts and vowing to be more loving, tolerant, and understanding. It may mean writing a half dozen letters of apology to people we have wronged or giving up the ill feelings we have for people who have wronged us.

I never did forgive my father until after his death. This is not the way to do it, because then grief at the time of death becomes more intense. A part of almost every grieving experience is the feeling of guilt. This may be over not having seen them before they died, not being there when they died, not having done all that we should have done before they died, or blaming ourselves for their death. Obviously, if we are alienated from the person who dies the guilt will be more severe. This was true in my case, and it continued until I forgave my father. You see, there was a part of me that said, "It's okay to be angry," and a part of me that said, "You are supposed to love your father," and I did. Because of the ambivalence, I felt guilty until I forgave him—even though I had to do it after his death. I had to verbally forgive him in the presence of God and another person so I could let go of the anger. I will never forget the personal release that I felt, and I experienced God's grace in a most meaningful way —peace of mind.

Don't con yourself

Making direct amends becomes even more difficult at times because there are some subjects we would like to avoid. It is no good to say to ourselves: "I admit that my relation with so-and-so is wrong, but I'll get over it. Time will take care of it." What a terrible con job we are doing on ourselves! Time will not heal a burst appendix nor will it heal a feeling of guilt or resentment. All of these need surgery—either physical or spiritual. Spiritual surgery requires the painful process of setting right our relationships with people. Neglect this surgery and the body may become sick and destroy itself physically, emotionally, or spiritually. This is not a threat, but a *reality.*

I am reminded of the man who was suffering from bleeding ulcers. He was filled with unresolved resentment toward many people who had hurt him throughout his life—people who had taken advantage of him, partly because he had allowed them to do it. However, he was unable to accept his part of the problem and refused to let go of his anger. Finally, surgery was required for his ulcer. He lost three-fourths of his stomach. Within a short time his ulcer returned and he was again finding blood in his stool. This unresolved resentment (and the ulcer) continued until he was found dead in his apartment. He had bled to death because he refused to resolve his anger by forgiving those people who had hurt him. He had refused to make amends.

Another way we con ourselves is by believing that we can get along without other people. Maybe there have been times in life when we have been hurt by others, and we come to the conclusion that the way to avoid this is to steer clear of people. It is true that many people are unlovable, vain, cruel, selfish, critical, and unsympathetic. But withdrawing from people is not the way to escape our need to make amends. The very fact that we are avoiding people probably means that we have not resolved some hurt or resentment. Also if we shut ourselves off from people, we shut ourselves off from God as well.

Often we feel like avoiding those who resent us. After all, who likes to be around an angry person? But maybe we need to hear what they have to say to us. This does not mean that we let them abuse us, but perhaps there is some truth behind their anger—otherwise they would not be angry. If we keep fleeing from people who might injure us, acting as though we are always the innocent ones, and complaining to God about how badly we are treated, we may never discover how we might have wronged them. In fact, we may only be using God as an escape from unpleasant experiences which could add to our character. Is not this partly what Jesus had in mind when he said: "Love your enemies and pray for those who persecute you" (Matthew 5:44)? This means that we are not to flee from them or resent them but forgive them, make amends, and be willing to listen to them. Without making amends we would not be able to love our enemies, because *the prerequisite for loving is forgiving*. Maybe this is why religion is sometimes referred to as "soft" and why some agnostics see it as an infantile attitude toward life, because we flee from our enemies and use our religion to escape life instead of using it to face life and love our enemies.

I remember a pastor friend of mine who was having difficulty in his parish. The people had taken one minute incident, removed it from its context, and blown it out of proportion. They also wanted to get rid of him because of his confrontive ways of dealing with people, but this had been concealed in the other accusation.

My friend had worked hard with these people and together they had accomplished much in the church. To have it all end this way was more than he could take. He began to isolate himself from his enemies in the congregation. One day he went out for a long walk in a wooded area near his home, which he had often done to get away by himself. As he left the road to enter the woods he heard the sound of footsteps behind him. He looked behind him but could not see anyone. He thought walking in the woods would allow him to be alone with God. He began to pray. Then he heard the footsteps again. He became so disturbed and frightened that he began to run along the path. He stopped two or three times to listen and each time he heard the noise of people walking behind him. He felt like a man pursued. He felt frantic and desperate. He recalled wanting so much to get away from people, and to find a refuge in God. But he continued to hear the feet. Finally he decided to sit down and face who or whatever it was. But no one came; the sound of the feet disappeared, and he heard God's voice within telling him that the feet were his and that the life that excludes people cannot find God either. Unless we feel that we deserve God's forgiveness because we have worked at making amends with people, the "peace which passes all understanding" will elude us.

Please do not misunderstand me. There are times when we must avoid certain people. We need to take time to be alone with God and it becomes necessary to shut out the demands of people and things. At times it is appropriate to use God as a refuge, a hiding place, a retreat, but then we need to go back to people and to our enemies, forgiving them in spite of their criticism, loving them in spite of their disapproval, but not needing to like their meanness, to trust their disloyalties, or to believe that they will make amends with us. Through this experience we can be strengthened and brought closer to God and perhaps even learn to serve him better because we were willing to pray for our enemies.

There are also times when we need to avoid other people because of their unwillingness to be reconciled with us. There is no benefit in allowing others to abuse us. This only enables them to be irresponsible and results in our martyrdom. Jesus tells us, "If anyone will not receive you or listen to your words, shake off the dust from your feet as you leave that house or town" (Matthew 10:14). Continuing to try to mend relationships with some people can be a waste of time and energy. And if we persist in setting ourselves up for hurt and rejection, we may need to examine why we do it. Perhaps it is because we think we need the forgiveness of these people in order to forgive ourselves. We don't! The only forgiveness we need is God's.

We might like to have the forgiveness of others, but we do not need it in order to forgive ourselves or for our own salvation.

Making amends means making things right with people; it means forgiving and loving our enemies; it means being alone with God at times but using him as a refuge *and a strength,* and it means returning to where life is lived after we have been alone with God. We need to get back out into the world. And because we have been with our Lord we are stronger, braver, better people than before.

Making amends with specific people is one of the most important aspects in helping with your healing!

> Making amends with specific people . . .
> Why, Lord?
> I'll get over it.
> Time will take care of it!
>
> But the negative thoughts don't go away . . .
> And the longer I wait
>   the more difficult it becomes.
> It's still there!
>
> And even worse—
>   they come out in ways that tell me
> I'm completely out of control,
>   leave me embarrassed and ashamed,
>   as well as feeling worthless and alone.
>
> Lord, give me the courage to make things right,
>   the grace to forgive my enemies,
>   the wisdom to be alone with you at times,
>   and the strength to continue working on my recovery.
>   Amen

10 Only One Day at a Time

Let us search and try our ways, and turn again to the Lord.　　　　　Lamentations 3:40

THE ONLY WAY THAT WE CAN continue to grow is to reflect daily on our behavior—on our assets and liabilities. Recovery is not a once and for all event; it is a process that must be worked at every day. Also recovery is not just being renewed or restored; it is much more encompassing than that. It speaks of the wholeness of a person, not just spiritual or relational health, but one's emotional and physical healing as well. And recovery implies the humanness of the individual, which presupposes that we make mistakes and fail daily. Therefore we need to work at our recovery every day.

In Chapter 8 we discussed five ways of becoming more aware of our unconscious—through talking, writing, recording our dreams, reflecting on our behavior, and meditation and prayer. The last two methods are particularly helpful. In this chapter we will be discussing the value of taking a daily personal inventory of our strengths and weaknesses so that we can fulfill our potential as a person. This way we can make better use of our assets and admit to our liabilities so that we can work at changing them.

In the first nine chapters (steps), the emphasis was on healing the past. Now that this has begun, we are ready to let go of our painful past and concentrate on the present. This does not mean that we will never discover other painful memories from our past that need healing, because we will. So we need to be open to that possibility, but by now we have probably finished with much of our past so that we can work on living today.

Taking a personal inventory every day could sound boring, especially if you only think of listing what we did wrong. Our daily reflection, however, must also include what we did right. Otherwise, we will never be able to work toward fulfilling our potential as a person. Of course, we need to be aware of our destructive life-style so that we know what needs to be changed and what limitations need to be accepted. Knowing what we can change and what we cannot change is vital to our recovery. Often people think that either they have to work at being perfect, or they have already arrived and have nothing left to do. We need to accept realistically that we have not arrived but are in the process, and also that we never will be perfect, except in eternity. The willingness to change what we can, and accept what we can't, has to be kept in tension every day by asking God for the wisdom to know the difference.

Continuing to look daily at our life-style could also be considered a drag if we do not realize that this results in a happier, fuller life. If we can anticipate this payoff, it might be easier for us to get into the habit of doing it daily. It can become like all of the other routine things that we do each day. When it becomes a part of us it will not seem stifling but liberating and exhilarating, because it becomes an opportunity for discovery and affirmation, as well as growth and maturity.

Continuing to take our inventory

There are at least four different ways to take a personal inventory. There is the inventory at the end of every day, the situational inventory following an anxiety-producing experience, the periodic times alone or with a trusted person(s), and the semiannual psychospiritual checkups.

As usual a few nights ago, before I went to bed, I reflected over how I had spent my day. I thought I had been more helpful than hurtful, more sharing than self centered, more honest with my feelings—like anger, love, fear, and joy, more active, doing things that resulted in good feelings, *but* aware that for some time—perhaps two or three years—I have not always been sure of my plan for the day. I know generally what things need to be done, but how they are going to happen I will not know until they happen. A few days ago, for example, I was to speak to a group on a particular subject. How it was going to come out I wasn't certain and didn't know until I had done it. Before, I would have had it all written out and been working on it for days. But it came out so easily. It flowed out as if it had all been done in advance. This does not mean I had not thought about it or become familiar with the subject, but I did not have it *all* planned out.

So it may be with many of the things that we do. When we have worked at our spiritual recovery for a while, whittled off some of the rough edges, and have the kind of

111

peace of mind which only God can give, we can let a lot of things just happen. Many times this is the way God works his wonders with us. We only have to be open enough to his leading. Many creative people have said that when they started a project they did not know where they were going with it or how it would end up. They may have had a general idea of what they wanted to do, but the result remained to be seen. It is like the potter beginning with a piece of clay and not knowing what the object will look like until it is finished. But a combination of skill and openness to God, others, and our environment allows the creative spirit to spring forth in us.

This is what I learned about myself the other day while taking my personal inventory—that my recovery had helped me to be more creative. But I also learned that to maintain that creativity, I had to continue my daily inventory. Otherwise, I might not keep what I had found. I might lose touch with the special creative seed God has planted in us all. We need to cultivate and nurture the little seedlings inside us, so that we can continue to unfold and expand—so new thought, enlightenment, and wisdom can come forth. We do not know what we will become, but I hope we will continue our daily inventory so we will know where we need to grow.

We need to keep in mind that it is okay even if everything doesn't come out right. There will be failures and dreams will dissolve. We will be left hanging and at loose ends. But we need to remember that there are opportunities here too. When we have situations that cause us to be disturbed, we need to evaluate what caused us to be upset. Was our self-worth threatened or did we feel obligated, guilty, or unnecessarily responsible? Were we feeling afraid, alone, or hurt? If we can understand why we felt or reacted the way we did, we can learn from it so that our responses become more appropriate and healthy.

Occasionally we need to spend time alone or with another person(s), and we also need to have an annual or semiannual checkup with a competent person who is devout, perceptive, and insightful. This could take the form discussed in Chapters 4 and 5—where we spend some time alone to take a moral inventory followed by discussing the issues which bother us with another trusted person.

Looking closely at specific crisis situations, spending time alone, and having a checkup from time to time help us to learn from our behavior. And our continued work with our inventory will be encouraged by the awareness that within us there is the still, small, creative force that is waiting to burst forth anew another day. We will recover by reflecting on what we do, responding to that creative spark within, and trusting God to guide the tiny flame inside us toward a more meaningful, happy life.

As your day is, so shall your recovery be

The story of Simon the Pharisee is a good illustration of a person who never really came to terms with himself (Luke 7:36-50). He was a man who was satisfied with himself, he had no need for forgiveness, and knew little about love. Jesus told him: "He who is forgiven little, loves little." Simon's trouble was his emphasis on living the law literally and his belief that he could find self-realization through that method.

We talked earlier in this chapter about the importance of realizing our potential. We are also aware of how destructive it is not to live up to our capacities. We are aware too that often the most creative people are those who have seen themselves as they are and through the process of reflection and daily inventory have found a sense of integration which results in peace of mind.

Achieving peace of mind, however, does not mean that we will be able to live without tension. In fact, to live without tension would mean that we are dead. Some tension is good; otherwise we might not be motivated to do anything. To pursue a tensionless life is like pursuing happiness—you will never reach the goal. Happiness and peace of mind are by-products of a meaningful life rather than goals in themselves. Usually real peace of mind does not come just from following rules or a tension-free situation, but from dedicating ourselves to something greater than ourselves and the completion of a creative task which often is filled with tension. Usually, a tensionless existence leads to frustration and a feeling of emptiness rather than peace of mind.

In the same sense, self-actualization is seldom achieved when it is sought directly. Like happiness and peace of mind, self-realization comes as a by-product. We realize our fullest potential when we commit ourselves to a task great enough to call forth all of our talents and abilities—not just keeping the law as Simon did. Simon was not aware that peace of mind was the result of fulfilling his potential through meeting the apparently overwhelming challenges of life. Similarly, some people could get so bogged down with their daily inventories that they stifle their creativity as well as their peace of mind.

Simon was a good man. He was a religious man, and like most religious people he had little sympathy or understanding for those who did not keep religious observances. Morality had become an end in itself and this was blinding him to really fulfilling his potential as a person. Through his preoccupation with avoiding sin, he had become unaware of the greatest sin—being out of relationship with people. This was evident in the way he rejected the "woman of the city" in the story.

This is one of the dangers of self-reflection. We can become so engrossed and preoccupied by our own progress, that we thwart the very progress which we desire. This is why it is important to do our inventory occasionally with other people and not just by ourselves. This way we will receive feedback from others who can see us more objectively than we can see ourselves. We will not "worship" the inventory process or our reflecting, but we will experience the peace of mind which is the result of our personal inventory.

I met a woman once who was having difficulty going to sleep, because she was "working" so hard at going to sleep. I also remember the man who was not able to have an orgasm, because the orgasm had become more important than the relationship and the process of loving and being loved by his spouse. Both of these situations were rectified when the attention was taken off attaining results and placed upon the process. When the woman stopped trying to sleep she found that she could. And when the man stopped concentrating on having an orgasm, he became successful. The "ends" were achieved because they became by-products of the "means."

Simon had thought that his primary concern was in personal fulfillment. He believed that this would give him meaning for life. Somehow he had not understood that a meaningful life required a commitment to something outside of himself. We all need to have a point of reference outside of ourselves—namely God. Meaning for life cannot be found through self-actualization but through responsible relationships with people and with God. It was this lack of personal responsibility in relationships for which Jesus criticized Simon. The pathway to personal maturity and the creativity to live up to our potential does not come from excessive self-actualization, but *commitment*—to God and to our neighbor.

One of the privileges that I had at the first parish I served was to help organize a senior citizens' group. It soon became the most dynamic group in the congregation. I am convinced that this happened because this organization filled a need for these people. Retired people often develop all kinds of illnesses to fill the vacuum of the empty hours unless new interests are discovered and old interests are reactivated. In the senior citizen organization as well as within the Christian church the concept of commitment is central—the commitment to a purpose, to others, and to God. We *find* our lives, not by holding on to them, not by jealously guarding them, but by freely giving them and by losing them in caring for others. As Jesus says: "Whosoever would save his life will lose it, and whoever loses his life for my sake will find it" (Matthew 16:25).

In addition to this, Simon's condemnation was not so much because he was not a good man as that his pattern of living stood in the the way of attaining the important values. Simon was responsible for his own life, but he didn't feel any responsibility to those around him. He was so preoccupied with keeping the moral law that he cut himself off from people. It was this behavior that prevented him from fulfilling his potential as a person and finding real meaning for his life.

Recovery from illness requires the same thing. It will never happen by spending all our time looking within. We need to look at our relationships and work at correcting whatever went wrong. It is true that this story of Simon is a good illustration of a person who never came to terms with himself, because he spent all his energy keeping the law. Consequently, he could not see any value in relationships and was not committed to others or to God. As a result, he had no point of reference by which to take his daily inventory in pursuit of his recovery.

Lord, we want so much to be happy!
We long for peace of mind.
But we forget that we lose it
  when we seek it.

Lord, help us to realize that
Recovery
  is a by-product of a life of self-evaluation . . .
  of being in relationship with you and others . . .
  and of responsible commitment which requires admission of
  wrongs.

Happiness and peace of mind are achieved
  when the means becomes more valuable than the end.
For if we will only save our own life
We will lose it.

Lord, help us to lose our preoccupation with ourselves
  as well as our tunnel vision . . .
So that we can find a more abundant life,
  and so recovery will not elude us.

Amen

11 Power to Do God's Will

> For God is at work within you, helping you want to obey him, and then helping you do what he wants. Philippians 2:13 LB

DURING THE WRITING OF THIS BOOK a very dear friend died of a heart attack. The last time we were together was more than three months before his death. He was a pastor in a large suburban congregation. The last attack was either the fourth or fifth he had had over the last few years. Only a few months earlier he and his wife had lost their oldest son.

Through the experience of losing my friend I was reminded again of the injustices and pain all around. I was also struck by the feeling of how useless and senseless his death was, because he was such a loving, compassionate, understanding man. I saw once more how some of us are so busy caring for others that we do not care for ourselves, and I realized how much we need the guidance and wisdom of God through meditation and prayer.

Sooner or later the pain and brokenness of the world catches up with us and then we discover how really helpless we would be without God. All too soon we experience hurt, fear, alienation, loneliness, and tension. Inevitably, we get broken and we bleed; our dreams crumble; our bodies age; the friends we once loved are no longer there. Though we will win in a million ways, all of us—some day —will end up losers. When that happens we cry out about the injustice as Job did: "Surely you cannot fail to see my innocence! Surely you see how I have behaved . . . Have I been a companion of falsehood or hastened my steps toward deceit?" (Job 31:4-6 NAB). Like Job, we may feel estranged and separated from God. We may feel our whole world has fallen apart and it can't be mended as simply as in the nursery rhymes of Jack and Jill. We have to do more than kiss the injured parts to make them heal. Real healing takes time, sometimes a long time—usually much longer than we anticipate. Unless we have the added dimension made possible through meditation and prayer, we will never recover spiritually, emotionally, and physically.

What is meditation and prayer?

There is a direct link between this chapter on meditation and taking a daily personal inventory in the previous chapters. This does not mean that they cannot be done separately, but I believe they are more productive when interwoven. The combination of reflecting on our behavior, and seeking God's will for our life and the power to carry it out, can be an aid to both steps. Unless we seek to change those things which we need to change, taking a personal inventory is a waste of time. And unless we have God's help we may not know what things we are able to change or have the courage to change them.

There is also a direct relationship between meditation and prayer. Prayer is raising our hearts and minds to God and in this sense it includes meditation. It may be in the form of words or as secret as a desire. It also has the same function as meditation and that is to get our will in tune with God's. Prayer, however, is a petition to God and usually follows meditation. This occurs because meditation opens the channel to God so that our prayers will become his will for us. After all, God knows our needs better than we know them ourselves.

Meditation is an art, not a science. Meditation is reflecting and creatively responding to God. There is no scientific method in this approach. Meditation is allowing the mind of God to break in upon us, and the purpose of prayer is the same—that our will should become God's will. This intent should color all of our prayer and meditation time (cf. Vernon J. Bittner, "Meditation," *Leadership Training School Program,* 1963, pp. 6-15).

Meditation can be thinking and reflecting on God's Word (or some other writing) and neither debating nor rejecting what God has to say to us. It is resting quietly and allowing God to speak to us through words. However, meditation may also be allowing God to speak to us directly through people and the environment around us.

Meditation cannot be imposed or forced. It is being relaxed enough to breathe deeply the grace and will of God without daydreaming. We need to begin with our goal in mind—to be in relationship with God so that we can draw nearer to the mind of God. Yet meditation is more like free association than direct thinking, because the latter becomes forced thought. Meditation must be "free"; otherwise it is not meditation.

But what happens if our mind wanders from the point

of meditation? When this occurs, we should not become disturbed, but realize that our thoughts will eventually return to the purpose of the meditation. This process can be illustrated by comparing it to the instincts of a homing pigeon. The pigeon when released far away from home may wander from its course, much as our thoughts may wander. However, since the goal is well set in the instinct of the bird, it will eventually come back to its course and find home. Much in the same way, without forcing, our minds will come back to our purposes in meditating, and within this atmosphere we can also be led naturally to hear what God has to say to each of us.

How to prepare for meditation

Preparation for meditation is one of the most important parts of meditation. No matter how short a period we may have for meditation, the first few minutes should be spent in preparing ourselves to speak with God. We must quiet our minds, our bodies, and our spirits.

One of the problems we may have in meditation is that we come rushing into God's presence with our minds full of conflicting thoughts. At this point we are too much out of breath, mentally and spiritually, to be able to speak with God, or to listen to his "still, small voice." The Psalmist said, "Be still, and know that I am God."

We need to be still, to stop all the thoughts that come rushing through our minds. We need to put aside the anxieties and fears that clamor for our attention. There are those who say, "Forget your anxieties and your fears and think about God." But this does not solve the problem. Those of us who have tried this method know that it does not. Often, we cannot get rid of anxious thoughts by thinking quiet thoughts. The only thing we may accomplish is to push the destructive thoughts into the subconscious mind. These return soon to haunt us in other ways—in being bored, being closed to God and not knowing why, being irritable and defensive, and being generally disinterested in meditation.

This does not mean, however, that just because we have found God we are always going to know the excitement of being close to him. There will be times when we are hurting in certain areas of our life and this affects our enthusiasm for life. Because we are human we need meaningful human relationships—and when those relationships are hurting it takes the edge off the meaningful relationship we seek with God.

How, then, do we quiet our minds? We need to identify why we are unable to quiet down. We must work at pinpointing what is disruptive so that it can be dealt with and we can go on to meditate. If this does not work, I would recommend that we start where we are and verbalize our feelings to God, as the psalmist did—and through the process cleanse ourselves so that we are open to God's will.

When we are free from the distractions, we can approach meditation with an open mind and a quiet spirit. Sometimes we may need to spend our entire meditation period becoming prepared, just as the psalmist did.

How do we meditate?

Now that our minds are open and our spirits are quiet, we are ready *to allow the mind of God to break in upon us.* Let this time and place belong to you and God—alone with each other.

Because meditation cannot be forced, we need to begin on a level of experience that is somewhat easy and not too demanding. We could begin with the miracle of the creation of nature or ourselves as human beings. From there we could move on to passages in Scripture—like the prayer our Lord told us to pray (Matthew 6:9-13). We might reread this prayer several times very slowly in order to absorb its deep meaning. Then we could go back and take one phrase at a time and concentrate on it.

Our Father . . . What does this mean for us? First, it says that because Jesus prayed this prayer, we have the guarantee that there is a Father—there is a God. Through the life, death, and resurrection of Christ we have the assurance that there is a God at work building his kingdom of mercy in a world that at times seems cruel, hard, and fatherless.

By saying "Our Father," Jesus was also acknowledging that God was there before he prayed. He is also saying that our Father knows what we need before we ask him (Matthew 6:8). Consequently it is not always as important that we know why we need to pray; it is more important that we *pray*. For in praying we will discover what we need, if we seek his will.

For example, when we go to a doctor we do not always know what we need. But the doctor most likely will know after he has examined the symptoms. So it is with our prayers to God. Often we will not know our deepest needs nor how to remedy them. But if we seek God's will for our lives we will find the answer—even though it may not be what we sought. Thank God that this is true—that he knows us before we pray and that his goodness is there before we come with our many words or with our long silences. This is why the most important aspect of prayer and meditation is that we enter into communion—into a personal relationship with God. This is why our *will* should emerge quite different from prayer and meditation than it was before we began. We come out reconciled, relying on God and surrendered to him. We come out willing to accept the good and the bad, because we believe that if we have his will in our life all things will work for good and we can say with childlike trust: "Not my will, but thine, be done."

By saying "Our Father," Jesus was saying too that he prays along with us and that we have the fellowship and support of other Christians. All of us who pray this prayer together are different, but we are all children of the heavenly Father. And when our prayers are weak or stupid, he lifts up our weak and ignorant words in his hands and helps us find the strength and the wisdom we need for life. In praying "Our Father," we are saying that we know he is present, he knows our needs, and he joins with us in one fellowship.

Once more we can read the prayer and again look at its inner significance. We can think of the man Jesus who first uttered this prayer, who became "the Word made flesh" and walked among us to teach and heal, who went to the cross to save, and who rose from the dead to redeem us. Then we can think of how the prayer begins with praise to God in heaven and ends with the praise of his kingdom, power, and glory.

Enclosed within our praise of God is all that we need. We pray for the acknowledgment of seeing God as God instead of having other gods or attempting to be our own god *(Hallowed be thy name)*. We pray that we will know the wonder of God in all his glory and power *(Thy kingdom come)*. We pray that his will become our will and the will of all people *(Thy will be done on earth, as it is in heaven)*. We pray for all of the things we need to sustain life—everything from the trivial to the spiritual *(Give us this day our daily bread)*. We pray, too, for the forgiveness of sins and the power to forgive others so that we will know his peace *(Forgive us our debts, as we forgive our debtors)*. We pray also that we will not reject our Lord and be lost to him *(Lead us not into temptation)*. And we pray that we will be kept free from the tyranny of the devil *(Deliver us from evil)*.

The Lord's Prayer is a total prayer. Within it are seven petitions that cover all of our needs. It can be prayed at the cradle and the grave. It can be spoken in great cathedrals and dark hovels. It never sends us away feeling empty or that it has not spoken our need. It is an example of a good prayer that we could use as a basis for meditation and as a model for our prayers.

What can we expect from meditation and prayer?

Perhaps one of the greatest rewards of prayer and meditation is the sense of belonging to God. Even though we feel alone, God is with us. We are no longer lost and without a purpose because we have God. We can see in him that there is truth, justice, and love in spite of the hostile world in which we live. We know that when we turn to him he will never leave us.

Through meditation and prayer we can discover God's will and mercy for us. We can use God as a mirror to see our own shortcomings. We will be able to determine what we can change and what we cannot change. We will have the courage to change what we can and the strength to accept what we cannot change.

For many, this may be their first attempt at combining a personal inventory with meditation and prayer. It may also be the first time that many have tried meditation. Do not be too disturbed if the first experience is not very fruitful. Begin bravely. God has promised if we earnestly seek him we will find him.

This may mean that even though we did not get anything out of the experience consciously, we will still get some good out of it. We do not need to get an emotional kick out of something in order for it to be worthwhile. Work at it. Remember, it needs to become a daily process because any good habit takes practice. Meditation and prayer can give you the opportunity to experience the closest relationship with God that you have ever known.

Through meditation and prayer we will want to think more like God thinks, we may want to talk to another person for more clarity and understanding, and we will want to spend more time talking with God because we have experienced his love—past, present, and future. Through meditation and prayer we can expect to find the serenity to aid in our healing.

Lord, it is good to know you are God.
It's good that you know what we are going to ask,
    before we ask it.
It's also comforting to know that we are not praying alone . . .
    for you pray with us.

Lord, help us to see you as God
    so that we can let you be that for us.
Grant that we will
    experience your mystery,
    enjoy the glory of your presence,
    and know the courage of your power.

Lord, may your will become ours . . .
May we attain what gives meaning and purpose to life.
Help us seek what we need for the good life . . .

not only what we need for physical and emotional health
but also what is necessary for spiritual health.

Lord, give us the good sense to confess our sins . . .
    so that we will know your forgiveness.
Give us the ability to accept it,
    because we have been forgiving as you have been forgiving.

Lord, we pray that we will have the wisdom never to reject you.
This will give us the strength to let you be God . . .
    so that we might know freedom instead of bondage,
    and communion instead of separation.

Amen

12 Give It Away or Lose It

Brethren, if a man be overtaken in any trespass, you who are spiritual should restore him in a spirit of gentleness. Look to yourself, lest you too be tempted.   Galatians 6:1

JUST BEFORE I STARTED WRITING this chapter I had a dream which I shared with my prayer group. As I began to talk about it I was not aware of its meaning or its specific relevance to writing this book. But as I talked about it I began to see not only how it applied to how this book would be received, but also to the emphasis of this last chapter— to share what I have found in Christ.

In my dream I found myself in the midst of a group of people who were agnostics. One of the individuals in the group was having difficulty finding any meaning for his life. In fact, he had become so despondent that he was nearly out of control. I wanted to reach out to him because I knew what that was like. I wanted to tell him that with God there was hope—if not for this life, certainly for the life to come. I wanted so much to give him the gift of hope so he could overcome his disappointments and begin to live.

But he was not a religious man and he had no identifiable religious resources. I did not think it would do any good to talk to him about my faith and my belief in eternal life. I felt helpless and frustrated. I was also confused and filled with conflict over what I should do—so I did nothing. This resulted in my feeling guilty for not trying—for not reaching out—even though my efforts might have fallen on deaf ears or been met with rejection.

After talking about my dream that day I realized that it not only spoke to the problem a lot of us have in sharing our faith, but it also expressed my anxiety about the acceptance of my work on the book for the past eighteen months.

One of the most difficult things for most of us to do is to share our faith—to share what we have found to be meaningful in our life—because we are afraid it will be unacceptable. We are fearful that what is dear to us will fall on deaf ears, closed minds, or hard hearts. However, unless we are willing to share our faith we will lose it. Our faith and our character are challenged and refined through the process of sharing. Through sharing we begin to grow in the fullness of Christ so that recovery, wholeness, and health can become a reality.

But how do we share our faith with others? In order to share our faith with others we need to act on the "spiritual awakening" that has taken place in our lives.

Having had a spiritual awakening...

There may be as many variations of spiritual awakenings as there are people. However, there are certain things in common. People gain confidence to do what they were not able to do before. They are more fully aware of who they are. Their lives seem to have a goal, instead of appearing to be only a dead end or something to be endured. They have been transformed, because they have found a source of power which they never realized before. They also possess more honesty, understanding, patience, humility, love, and peace of mind than they thought was possible. They have received the free gift of God's presence in their lives because they were ready to receive it.

Unless we have experienced this spiritual awakening, we are unable to reach out to others. This is the problem with many who are recovering—they have not been open to receive their Lord so they have nothing to share. The reason people refuse to witness to their faith is because they are spiritually bankrupt. However, sometimes they do not discover what they have until they risk passing it on.

I hope that I have not hurt anyone by saying this, but we must be honest with ourselves. Maybe this is the problem for many of us who are hesitant to share our faith. Maybe we really have not taken anything from our contact with our Lord that is worth passing on. Why? Because we have been closed to his love.

What has been your experience with Christ? Is it a vague sort of religious sense—admitting that there is a God, an inspired Bible, a historical person by the name of Jesus whose teachings and healing are admirable and whose personality is lovable—or is it Christianity? Are we really committed to him and his way of life? I hope we are, so that we can enter more fully into a living experience with Christ that will continue to change our life.

If our experience with Christ is somewhat vague, then we will have little to pass on. But if we have been touched by Christ, we cannot help but share it with others, no matter how fearful we are or how hard it may be to find a way. In one way or another, we will convey what we have found in Christ, hoping others will receive him too.

At our hospital we have a Share and Care group composed of terminal cancer patients and families who find strength in sharing their hurts and caring for each other. After meeting several months with this group, I found that patients and their families received support from each other because they realized there were others like them. They were strengthened to face their own situation by reaching out to each other. They spent time discussing their feelings of helplessness, everyday physical problems, questions about life and death, the quality of life, the importance of family support, and their faith in God or lack of it. By sharing their experiences, frustrations, and faith, these patients and their families found a strength and a power in each other and in God that they did not know existed for them.

There are all kinds of self-help groups like this which have discovered one great mutual benefit which Christ and the Christian church have valued for centuries—we are strengthened not only by the faith of others, but also by sharing our own. *If we do not share it we will lose it* and if others will not share it with us we will not find it. And having had an experience of finding Christ years ago and not doing anything with this discovery since then is not good enough. If that is the case we will be pretending that all is well, when all the while our experience is no longer living and vital.

We must take this matter of sharing our faith with others seriously. None of us is fully won to Christ unless we are using the gift God has given us to reach out, touch others, and bring them into the experience of newness of life. To possess this joy and serenity and not share it is selfish and unthinkable. I shudder to think what would have happened if the early church had done that. But regardless of the importance of others knowing about the love of Christ, we need the experience of carrying this message of hope and love to someone else so it becomes more dear to us.

For me as for you, there is risk involved in making a decision to share what we have found in Christ. For me and for many others I have known, doing something for God (such as telling another person what Christ means to me) means allowing the "still, small voice" to win out over the doubting or unwilling part of us. When we do not hear the small voice within us, it is usually because we are afraid to risk anything for God. We do not want to risk rejection, failure, or hurt to share our faith.

I mentioned earlier in this book that I have decided to follow my hunches on decisions I have to make each day, whether it be in the treatment of a client or in any contract I make with individuals in my everyday life. I feel that when I respond to the positive impulse of the moment, I am listening to the voice within me, and I have found that 9 times out of 10 it turns out right. And when it does not I have to remember that I am subject to human failings and at least I did my best.

But there is one factor that we do not take into account when we fail to risk doing things for God, and that is *God*. We forget that he has a purpose in what he calls us to do, and he knows all about our "feeble knees and the hands that hang down," and he is standing in the wings waiting to complete the work we have started when we took the risk! His part is to supply the "spirit of gentle persuasion" —the convincing power, the loving beckoning, the irresistible pull—and the openness and receptiveness in those we are trying to reach. Without that, neither you, nor I, nor the most dedicated Christian could hope to accomplish anything for God.

Our part, then, becomes easier as we trust the voice within, act on our positive impulses, and leave the results up to him. The finished work need not surprise us, embarrass us, concern us, or even be noticed by us. In one way it compares to building a house—the operator of the bulldozer seldom sees what gets built in the excavations he makes. All we need is a desire and a willingness. Sharing depends on our willingness to reach out with faith in God's help.

A few months ago a man in his early thirties came to me. He had become so depressed he was not functioning. He was married and had two children. Within the past few years, he had had a series of disappointments. He had lost several jobs, some as a result of the company folding and some because he was not selling his quota. Since college he had been working as a salesman, but had never really been happy doing it.

I asked him if there had ever been a time in his adult life when things were good for him. He told me that it was when he was working with a youth group in his church in Iowa. Since then things had gone downhill. His company had folded and he moved on. Things had become so bad that now he was bitter at God and had stopped going to church.

I asked him if he had ever considered the ministry. He was somewhat shocked to have me ask the question, but indicated that he had. It was during the time he was in Iowa. He had gone to speak to leaders of the church there and they told him there were no openings at that time in the Episcopal Church. He decided that the risk was too great to spend another four years going through seminary training and then not be sure of finding a position. Unfortunately, after making that decision things began to go bad for him. Not only did he lose a series of jobs and become very depressed but he lost his faith.

I told him he needed to get back to church whether he felt like going or not, and he must forgive God. I also suggested he think about the possibility of going to the seminary or find some other way of serving the church. It was obvious to me that Christ had meant a great deal to him once and because he stopped sharing that experience he lost the joy he once had.

About two weeks later he came back. There was a sparkle in his eyes and he seemed to have come alive. His downcast appearance and his depression were gone. This is the gist of what he said: "I found Christ again! I took your advice and went back to church. He had been there all the time, but I had been closed to him through my disappointments and bitterness.

"Just last week an acquaintance of mine asked me to come and help with their young people at church. I was hesitant but I went. I think I enjoyed myself more than I have for years. It was like my experience in Iowa. When you told me that my faith had died not only from my bitterness, but also because of not sharing it, I didn't believe you. I thought that it was true for others, but not me. But the other night I found out it was true. I was asked by one of the young adults what Christ meant to me. I told him. I can only say that it helped me tremendously and it gave me an exhilarating feeling. Now I know without a doubt that to reach out to others as Christ reaches out to us, is not only showing our colors, but it strengthens our faith and deepens our experience with him."

He had discovered the truth in a very hard way. He had to become totally depressed to discover how important it is to share his faith. I wonder how many others there are who are stuck in their recovery process because they are afraid and unwilling to share their faith? I'm sure there are many. If only they knew how rewarding it is to share their faith with others! To see the eyes of men and women begin to sparkle as they move from darkness into light, to watch their lives become filled with new purpose and meaning, to be aware of families being reunited, and above all to see people awaken to the presence of a loving God in their lives—these are things we experience if we are willing to share our faith with others!

There are some, of course, who would like to avoid sharing their faith by saying that they either have no talents or there is nothing for them to do. This is just an excuse. There is something for everyone to do and no one is without talents.

There will also be some disappointments in reaching out to others. There will be those who reject us and what we have to offer. When this happens we may question our ability to help others. Even though it is important to look at the way we approach people, making sure that we show concern, understanding, and a willingness to listen, we should not necessarily take their rejection personally. I know how hard this was for me to learn. I remember how anxious I was to do a good job when I first came to North Memorial Medical Center. I felt that I had to prove to the medical community my importance and value in the healing process. This not only put a lot of pressure on me and caused me to appear defensive at times, but resulted in my setting myself up as God because I was trying to be "all things to all people." This was okay until I received criticism for not being the super-chaplain I thought I should be.

This practice came to a screeching halt one evening when I was sitting at home. I began having chest pains as well as pains shooting up my arms toward my heart. I had all the symptoms, I thought, of a heart attack. I went back to the hospital and had an electrocardiogram. The examination indicated that I was not handling my stress very well. But that was not the only problem; I was taking rejection too personally because of my need to be perfect. I had to accept the fact that I was okay and that I did not need to be accepted by everyone—even Jesus did not have the luxury of that.

Another way to avoid disappointment in reaching out to others is not to become too highly elated when we have been successful in helping others, so that we take the credit that belongs to them or to God. The truth is that we would not be able to help anyone if they were not willing to be helped. Nor would we be able to help people who refused to be open to God's power in their life. And even more important, unless we are open to God's will, we will not have the power to help those we can help, the wisdom to know which ones we cannot help, and peace of mind to accept reality.

This does not mean that we should not feel good about helping others. Unless we get some rewards for helping others, we will probably stop doing it. What is important is to feel good about how we have helped, but realize that without God's power and the desire of the person to be helped we could do nothing. This way we also will not take all the blame if the person does not change.

Finally, disappointments in helping others can also be avoided if we do not become so personally involved that we become possessive of these people or give too much advice. If we do this we are taking too much responsibility for their recovery and we will feel hurt and rejected if they do not change. We must realize that we cannot manage or control anyone's life. We will regret it if we attempt to do this. Not only will they resent us for trying to run their lives, but they will blame us if things do not work out. Either way we lose. The only way sharing can become a "win" proposition for us, and those with whom we share, is if we have an objective concern for them. In this way we will show them that we do care *for* them, but we are unwilling to take care *of* them.

In the long run, however, sharing what we have found in Christ is rewarding, necessary, and a vital part of the recovery process. Unless we do this we will not find the serenity to practice what we have learned when we have to face the difficulties of life.

Putting the principles into practice

What we have been discussing throughout this book is a life-style. Recovery and being responsible for our own health involves a holistic pattern of living. It is hanging on to the joy and serenity that only Christ can give, whether we have failure or success. It is being able to adjust to life without despair or pride. It is the ability to accept poverty, sickness, loneliness, and grief with courage. It is the willingness to find contentment with the humbler, more durable satisfactions, when the flashy, superficial achievements elude us. It is not letting indifference over temporary successes lull us into thinking that we no longer need to share what we have found. It is transforming the calamities of life into assets, and opportunities for maturity and comfort to ourselves and those around us.

Some years ago, when I was still serving a parish, I received a call to come to a member's home. I knew that Harriet had a drinking problem and for some time her children had been trying to get help for her.

When I arrived, I could sense the tension of the family. Harriet was crying and was very angry. She was unable to understand why her younger daughter was unwilling to allow her to take care of the grandchildren. Her other daughter was attempting to explain that she could not trust her with the children because of her drinking.

I could tell that maybe this was the crisis that Harriet needed to decide to do something about her drinking. Previously the family had not even been able to get her attention. Now she was willing to hear that she had a drinking problem and that her family expected her to do something about it. She agreed not to drink any more that day and came to my office the next day.

The following morning I received a call from her telling me that she was not going to come. The only thing that I said to her was: "It is up to you . . . but the only person you are going to hurt by not coming is yourself." For Harriet, coming to see me was one of the most difficult decisions she had ever faced. At last she decided to come.

Our first session together would be called in Alcoholics Anonymous circles a "Fifth Step." Not only did Harriet admit to being drunk for 35 years and forgetting how to cook, among other things, but she talked about details in her life that she had been trying to drown for years. She spoke of her unhappy marriage, her adultery, and how she finally stopped denying her drinking problem when her own daughter refused to allow her to babysit her grandchildren.

There were many tears and prayers during that hour. But as the result of her confessions and knowing that I had forgiven her in the name of Jesus Christ, she experienced peace and serenity such as she had never known before. This was the beginning of her recovery from alcoholism. I had several more sessions with her, some with her husband present. Unfortunately, her husband didn't live very long to enjoy the transformation that took place in her life. But he did see her begin the process.

In spite of her husband's death, she began to put into practice the recovery principles she had learned, even though she never went to Alcoholics Anonymous. In most cases people are not able to get their life together without the help of AA, but she began the recovery process by turning her life over to God. During a serious illness that followed her husband's death, she continued to make amends with the people she had harmed.

After recovering from her physical illness she began to share what she had found in Christ. When she had the opportunity she told others of her problem and what peace she had found in her Lord. In spite of her age, meager income, poor health, and loneliness, she wanted to serve others in whatever way she could. She called on people in nursing homes, visited those who were confined to their homes, and initiated the formation of an intercessory prayer group. She had found contentment in loving and serving others as she had been loved and served. She was sharing what she had found. God had helped her to transform her life and she wanted others to know that joy, too. And she knew that she was going to have to practice what she had found each day of her life or she would lose it. This, too, was a part of helping with her healing.

Fifteen years later Harriet suffered a very serious heart attack. I was called to her room. She was very weak. I could tell that her age had taken its toll. She was now 79, but she still had that twinkle in her eye and that serenity she had found.

Yet there was something different about her. Her life seemed more fulfilled, and she appeared to have a sense of completeness. It was as though she were ready to let go of her life here for something else that she believed was better.

We talked for only a few seconds, and then she asked if I would read her favorite parable. I knew exactly what it was, because we had shared it before. It was the parable of the lost sheep—it was dear to her because it exemplified her life. She, too, had been lost, but had been found. She had strayed from the love of God and her family, but had come back because God had helped her be open and experience love and forgiveness. Even more, she was willing to reach out to others, that they might be found and experience God's joy and peace in their lives. She also knew how exhilarating and strengthening it was for her to help others know God's healing and wholeness. I will never forget that experience with Harriet and her son and daughter-in-law. She had looked at me, smiled, and said, "Do something for me. Read—my story."

What do you think? If a man has a hundred sheep, and one of them has gone astray, does he not leave the ninety-nine on the mountains and go in search of the one that went astray? And if he finds it, truly, I say to you, he rejoices over it more than over the ninety-nine that never went astray. So it is not the will of my father who is in heaven that one of these little ones should perish. (Matt. 18:12-14)

Before I had finished, she had fallen asleep. We stood by the bed for some time. There were tears of sadness, but there were many more tears of joy, for she had been lost and had been found—and she had shared the joy she had found with others.

Shortly, she woke up and whispered "It's all right." Then Harriet died. But she had experienced God's healing in her life. She had known the joy of spiritual recovery, and she had helped with her healing by sharing it with others.

Lord, the only love we keep is the love we give away!
It is only in sharing our faith
   that we will keep it!
For if we refuse to give it away
   we will lose it.

Help us to have the good sense to give it away—
   so that it doesn't die within us,
   so that we do not despair,
   so that you are not dead to us, and
   so that life does not become meaningless!

"For whoever would save his life
   will lose it,
And whoever loses his life for my sake
   will find it."
Lord, help us to find your love by sharing it with others.

                                      Amen

A
Final
Word

CARING FOR OUR OWN HEALTH or working on our spiritual recovery is difficult, and it is something that we have to work at every day. There will be days when our lives will glow because we are filled with the power of God. And there will be days when we may feel abandoned by God. But we need to commit ourselves to keep on reaching out for God's comforting and strengthening hand. Unless we do this, healing and spiritual recovery will elude us. Spending eternity with God is a gift. But the salvation which Jesus talked about is something that we can experience in the present as well as the future, if we are willing to be dedicated to our own spiritual, emotional, and physical health through the process of spiritual recovery.

May God help us to commit ourselves to spiritual growth and the willingness to share it with others that we might know the joy of healing and recovery now.

You can help with your healing.

A Note to Readers:

Living the Christian life is a lifelong process. We begin to grow when we courageously look at our limitations and through God's strength deal with them in a constructive way. To help in this process, *You Can Help with Your Healing* has reinterpreted the twelve steps of Alcoholics Anonymous in light of the Christian faith. If you found this book helpful, you might be interested in doing an in-depth study on it, either privately or in a group. This can be done using a prepared Study Guide, also available from Augsburg Publishing House. The Study Guide aids readers in adapting the twelve steps to their daily living. Here are the Twelve Steps for Spiritual Living contained in the Study Guide:

1. We admit our need for God's gift of salvation, that we are powerless over certain areas of our lives and that our lives are at times sinful and unmanageable.
2. We come to believe through the Holy Spirit that a power who came in the person of Jesus Christ and who is greater than ourselves can transform our weaknesses into strengths.
3. We make a decision to turn our will and our lives over to the care of Christ as we understand him—hoping to understand him more fully.
4. We make a searching and fearless moral inventory of ourselves—both our strengths and our weaknesses.
5. We admit to Christ, to ourselves, and to another human being the exact nature of our sins.
6. We become entirely ready to have Christ remove all of these defects of character that prevent us from having a more spiritual life-style.
7. We humbly ask Christ to remove all of our shortcomings.
8. We make a list of all persons we have harmed and become willing to make amends to them all.
9. We make direct amends to such persons wherever possible, except when to do so would injure them or others.
10. We continue to take personal inventory and when we are wrong, promptly admit it, and when we are right, thank God for his guidance.
11. We seek through prayer and meditation to improve our conscious contact with Christ as we understand him, praying only for knowledge of his will for us and the power to carry that out.
12. Having experienced a new sense of spirituality as a result of these steps and realizing that this is a gift of God's grace, we are willing to share the message of his love and forgiveness to others and practice these principles for spiritual living in all our affairs.

You may purchase copies of the Study Guide (10-7414) for *You Can Help with Your Healing* from: Augsburg Publishing House, 426 S. Fifth Street, Box 1209, Minneapolis, MN 55440.